FINDING
your
BALANCE

*Caring of Mind,
Body and Soul in
Times of Discomfort,
Instability and Surgery*

FINDING *your* BALANCE

*Caring of Mind,
Body and Soul in
Times of Discomfort,
Instability and Surgery*

KATE S. O'SHEA

INSTITUTE OF ORTHOPEDIC PSYCHOLOGY
SAUSALITO, CALIFORNIA

First printed February 1995
10 9 8 7 6 5 4 3 2 1

Illustrations by Natalie Roth and Kate O'Shea
Cover design by Abigail Rudner, On the Wave Visual
  Communications
Tree of Life logo by Natalie Roth
Book design by Jerald Volpe
Typesetting by the BOOKWORKS

Printed in the United States of America

Library of Congress Cataloging-in-Publication Data
O'Shea, Kate S., 1955—
    Finding Your Balance

    Includes bibliographical references, index

                              94-096423
ISBN 0 9642676-9-1

The Institute of Orthopedic Psychology
P.O. Box 3178, Sausalito, CA 94966.

To my clients, who have given me the gift of their trust and the honor of accompanying them on their path.

Acknowledgments

This book could not have reached its wide audience without the generosity of Mrs. Muriel Flanders. My deepest gratitude, with the hope that many lives will be touched.

I have had extraordinary guides and companions along my path. It is hard to express the depth of my thanks for their contributions to my life, but here goes:

Dr. Rodrick Turner of Boston gave me the opportunity to come this far with his surgical mastery. I'm so glad that he took the risk, trusting his skill and my commitment to thrive.

My teachers and mentors are brilliant women who taught me to think critically, expand my perspective, honor the power and mystery of the human spirit, and express my creativity through my work. Listed in the order they came into my life: Anna Marie Sandler, Kerstin Lindley-Jones, Marie Smith, Judith McKinnon, Louis Barrie, Joyce Riveros and Anita Feder-Chernilla. Many thanks to my colleague Diana Sloat, advanced Eutony student, who introduced me to Joyce Riveros.

Love and blessings to my parents Phyllis and Chuck O'Shea for a lifetime of unconditional love that has made me strong, to Herb Isenberg for his loving encouragement and to my dear small friends RC and Huey, who supplied their constant love and comic relief throughout my hours of writing – and not writing.

The process of writing has its own family:

Deep appreciation to Nancy Anderson who served as editor and midwife for this project. Her wise guidance of when to push and when to relax made it possible for me to bring my inner experience into the world.

My clients who shared their stories with me and allowed me to bring their experiences into print. (Names and circumstances have been changed for the sake of privacy.)

Insightful commentary on my early drafts was made by Helen Strodl, Phyllis O'Shea, Jan Venolia, Mili Kari, Shirley Davalos, Elizabeth Beach and Herb Isenberg. The breadth of their perspectives enriched me and the book. Patricia Parker acted as my personal reference librarian, model for the Chapter Seven illustrations and intellectual buddy.

Natalie Roth provided the illustrations in Chapter 7. Her self-knowledge informs the drawings with a quality I had only hoped to achieve. Jerald Volpe brought life to the book's pages with his simple but elegant design. Abigail Rudner created the luminous cover.

Early support for this project from David Cheek, M.D. and William Stewart, M.D., convinced me that the medial community needs to hear my perspective. Wink Franklin, at the Institute of Noetic Sciences, provided encouragement and support in the final days of the process making the finish line easier to reach.

Extra special thanks to Helen Strodl, of Cheshire Cat Books in Sausalito, for her infinite patience, support and wisdom as she listened to detail after detail of wording and book design.

Finally, honor must be given to the thousands of laboratory animals who have sacrificed their lives, enabling humans to uplift our understanding and appreciation for the divine intricacies of the body. May we use their gift to the highest good for all beings and may we learn to use alternative models to eliminate all experimental uses of animals. Toward this goal donations can be sent to the American Fund for Alternatives to Animal Research, 175 W. 12th St. #16-G, New York, NY 10011-8275

Foreward

It was with great pleasure and excitement that I read *Finding Your Balance.*

Kate O'Shea overcame tremendous obstacles and soared. This book is the fruit of her accomplishments. It is also a step by step guide to the healing process, which is sometimes somatic, at other times psychological, but always a spiritual quest for wholeness.

Knowledgeable, well-meaning people have written "how to" books that are technically excellent. However, Kate's book has the added luster that can only come from understanding gleaned through the interior process of transforming the kinds of challenges she describes. Our need for alchemy in relation to our consciousness and our healing takes a guide who has accomplished this goal. Kate is such a person.

Having first met Kate as a student in my massage certificate class nearly 20 years ago, I can attest to her great physical improvements. When I think back to her limited mobility and difficulty in gait, I remember the struggles she had developing a grounded, balanced stance for giving massage. To see her now, after many years, walk up the stairs to my school with scarcely a hint of the former difficulty in movement is both astonishing and heartwarming.

Did this happen over night? No, there are no miracles of that sort. To even think in that vein is to court disappointment. However, what can happen is through a slow, determined process of learning we can use ourselves better and better. The hand of our consciousness can gently and constantly direct and redirect our efforts until we more easily hold our growth. We must come to a place of psychological and spiritual peace with the struggle. We must embrace our work, as defined in *Finding Your Balance*, as a way of life. It must permeate our thinking and consciousness at all levels.

It sounds like an enormous task, but with the right attitude it can be fun. It is inspiring to know that you can improve what life has given you. This book and this woman give hope and a methodology for attaining that goal.

– Judith McKinnon
Oakland, California

Judith McKinnon, Founder and Director of the McKinnon Institute, has taught professisonal massage and bodywork since 1973. She has served as a gubinatorial appointee to the state Physical Therapy Examining Committee, taught internationally since 1984 and contributed widely to advancing the field of therapeutic massage and bodywork in health care.

CONTENTS

ILLUSTRATIONS

About this Book

THIS BOOK WAS WRITTEN TO NOURISH YOUR EXPERIENCE of surgery and other trauma, and to help you go beyond the conventionally accepted level of recovery. It shows you, the "patient," how to build dignity and participate actively throughout your recuperation and maintenance. It also provides a window for loved-ones and care-givers who wish to more deeply understand the experience of those recovering from physical challenges. My experience is primarily with orthopedic problems, however, I believe the insights presented here will be useful to anyone who has undergone surgery, trauma, or simply wants to develop a more comfortable and aware relationship with their body.

When I was 10 years old I had my second of four orthopedic surgeries to correct a congenital hip disorder. I received a get well card that looked like a computer key punch card addressed "to someone who has been spindled, folded and mutilated." Today, many of my clients feel similarly chewed up in the medical system. They feel rushed, their concerns often trivialized. A feeling of alienation from one's own body is not uncommon. The busy world we live in can make us feel that taking time to heal is unimportant or a sign of weakness. There seems to be something threatening to the status quo about the natural need to rest and recover. In truth, the time and attention given to healing is a wise investment in your long-term comfort and health. The time I spent learning to care for my body and its sensitive nature led to an inner friendship that will never end.

My desire to achieve physical comfort and freedom from the after-effects of surgery revealed my inner strengths and introduced me to remarkable people. The dynamic relationship between my mind and body proved to be undeniable. The more I learned about that relationship the more comfortable, active and resilient I grew. I have been a Bodywork professional for over 15 years, using my personal and professional training. My insights have helped my clients and, in turn, can help you shorten your time of discomfort, enriching your recovery and your life. Like me and my clients, you will learn the practical benefits of slowing down, being gentle with yourself and listening to the inner voice that is often overruled. Recovery, in the deep and lasting sense, means that you are a new person as result of the healing process. You can be more balanced than the person you were before facing the trauma. This book can help you learn how to maintain this new perspective, your body and mind meeting the challenges of life together.

How to use this book

It is most beneficial to read the chapters of this book in order. The ideas and stories presented in the early chapters prepare you to make best use of the tools offered later. Take time to absorb the insights and inspirations that emerge as you read. Chapters Four through Seven provide specific ways to put your new awareness into practice, increasing your comfort, mobility and peace of mind.

I use personal examples and client case histories to show how focusing attention within can have practical, lasting benefits. This focus will enable you to get to know and appreciate parts of yourself you may have been avoiding. You may begin to notice how your body can express metaphors for the themes in your life. I use my personal stories a great deal because I know my own inner processes best. My hope is that you will be inspired to explore your own inner life, finding your own insights and solutions. Attention, practiced patiently, allows you to take better care of yourself because you will be able to notice, interrupt and alter previously unconscious habits that contribute to discomfort. You become a more active participant in your health – and your whole life.

Audio and video tapes are available to enhance and expand on the tools presented in the book. See the Resources Section.

Begin with Awareness

This book is educational material, designed to provide introductory information. Before using any of this information you should make sure that it is appropriate to your body and your condition by consulting your doctor or other licensed health practitioner.

Not all programs are suitable for every individual. This or any other program could result in injury to you if it is not appropriate to your health and physical condition, or if it is not properly used and followed.

By using suggestions made in this book you assume the responsibility for making that decision, with your doctor or practitioner's advice, and you assume the risk of any injury or disability.

The author, the publisher and any party distributing this book are not responsible for any injuries, damages or losses which may arise from or in connection with the use of this book or the exercises or suggestions contained in it. They specifically disclaim any such liability. If while performing any of the exercises, you experience dizziness, pain, or any other unusual physical symptoms cease the activity until you have checked with your doctor or practitioner.

Your health is your responsibility and you assume all risk for it. This responsibility also gives you the power to make positive change in your life.

Orthopedic Psychology

ORTHOPEDIC PSYCHOLOGY IS AN EVOLVING FIELD DEDICATED to the study of consciousness as it expresses, and is expressed by the condition and functioning of the skeletal system and its related structures. *Finding Your Balance* presents a broad discussion of how our dynamic system of awareness and anatomy can be activated for health and well being. The Institute of Orthopedic Psychology is a center for education and research. The Institute can be contacted at P.O. Box 3178, Sausalito, CA 94966.

Chapter 1

A Question of Balance

Mr. Duffy lived a little distance from his body.

– James Joyce
"A Painful Case", The Dubliners

IF YOU ARE LIKE MANY PEOPLE, YOUR EXPERI-
ENCE with conventional medical practitioners
feels out of balance, as if something is missing. You
are right, there *is* something missing. Health care in
America has grown up under a system that prizes the
scientific method above all else. The body has been
separated from the humanity of the individual. Most
medical people are thoughtful and do their best to
give personal care, but are engulfed by the crush of
time and professional conventions. As "patients," we
learn to ignore our inner selves from the medical system's example. This is a great tragedy. We doubt our
ability to improve our own condition, relying on pills
and doctors to "fix" us. This book teaches you how

to become more knowledgeable about yourself, giving you tools to bring yourself back into balance. To begin, a little history will help explain how this systemic imbalance got started.

The mind-body problem in Western culture

The root of the problem is the long standing scientific belief that the mind is separate from the body. Four centuries ago, the ideas of philosopher and mathematician René Descartes led to the scientific revolution that separated the body from the mind. According to Descartes, and those who followed his ideas, the body was a machine, unaffected by the mind. This belief was a reaction against the extremes of medieval superstition and religious dogma which stressed unquestioning subservience to a wrathful God. It was a world with little rational order. Scientists like Descartes attempted to look at life apart from the subjective and irrational ideas of the time. Unfortunately, an overly scientific position, as with many corrections, went too far. Priests and wise women, once the healers of the community, were ostracized from the treatment of illness. Their spiritual and emotional perspectives – so necessary for well-being – were lost to the seductive pull of "progress."

Dr. William Stewart, Medical Director of the Program in Medicine and Philosophy at California Pacific Medical Center, refers to this artificial split of the body and mind as the "wound of Descartes." The unnatural division between our physical, mental, emotional and spiritual selves contributes to the fear and alienation in our present society. Without true connection to our physical selves, we feel lost in the world: estranged from our own core physically, emotionally and spiritually. Conventional medical practices encourage the surrender of our physical selves to a system that assumes to know more about our own well-being than we do, thus, creating a new god to place over ourselves. This "religion" has been in place so long that most people believe that they have no role in their own health. Just as Descartes questioned a system that was out of balance, it is time to question the outmoded authority in order to heal this wound.

The perspective of this book

My approach to health through awareness and movement has a feminine genealogy. It is decidedly different from the conventional, aggressive stance of our medical system and popular culture. This approach is the Feminine Principle in action: receptivity, the ability to listen and wait, respect for the subtlety of individual experience, nurturing of tiny awarenesses into fully expressed strengths. The experience of modern medicine can be like encountering the sharp point of a sword, cold and precise. While this masculine approach has given us the wonders of technology, it has also left us alienated from our humanity. The warm and gentle hand of the mother is needed to create balance.

I trace my professional influences to two women who developed their own schools of movement and awareness education when they were turned away as untreatable by the medical profession. Elsa Gindler[1] was diagnosed with tuberculosis in *1910* and was told to live out her days quietly in a sanitarium. Gerda Alexander[2] was born in *1908*. When rheumatic fever left her with a weakened heart, her doctors told her to marry a wealthy man and expect to live in a wheelchair. Neither accepted their prescribed fate. Each flourished through meticulous attention to their natural inner processes, discovering that within the quiet of the body lies a wealth of resources.

The importance of Gindler and Alexander's work is demonstrated by the wide influence they have had over the past 60 years in the fields of education, the arts, rehabilitation and the human potential movement, primarily in Europe. Both women were from Germany, where in the early 1900's there was great interest in bringing music and natural movement into education. Gindler and her students went on to bring body awareness and movement into the treatment of emotionally disturbed and disabled children and adults. Charlotte Selver, developer of the "Sensory Awareness" school in the U.S., was Gindler's student. Marion Rosen, Physical Therapist and founder of The Rosen Method of Bodywork, studied in Germany with a Gindler student in the 1930's. She brought the European approach to California. During 30 years of work as a physical therapist, she observed that people who talked with her got better faster. She combined this awareness with her European training to formulate her own method. I was one of the first Certified Rosen Practitioners.

Gerda Alexander first became a teacher of the Dalacroze Eurythmic Education, a method focused on experiencing music with the whole body. Later she founded her own system, Eutony, which emphasizes the development of total awareness of one's living anatomy in all aspects of life. Eutony is taught throughout western Europe, and in parts of Canada, South America, and in the United States. I studied Eutony for 3 years with Alexander's former assistant, Joyce Riveros. I am strongly influenced by Eutony principles of expanding awareness of the skin and skeleton, as a means for increasing balanced muscle tone and achieving ease in movement. This perspective is most helpful in moving with comfort and grace, even after surgery, injury or stroke.

The methods of Gindler, Alexander, and many other gifted teachers are now placed under the broad umbrella "bodywork." The following definition is the best I have found to describe this growing professional field:

> *"Bodywork...is a kind of sensorimotor education, rather than a treatment or procedure in the sense common to modern medicine...In this educational experience...the bodyworker is not "fixing" the client...the bodyworker is not an interventionist: s/he is a faclitator...touching hands are like flashlights in a darkened room. The "medicine" they administer is like self-awareness, and for many of our painful conditions, this is the aid that is most needed."*[3]

The consistent message throughout the schools that emerged from pre-war Germany, as well as other body-awareness oriented disciplines, is that you can improve your physical functioning through careful attention and patience. It is a simple prescription, yet one that requires new levels of self observation and discipline. Happily, the benefits are well worth it.

Many are searching

I am not alone in my search for answers to compliment conventional medical treatment. A Harvard University study, published in the New England Journal of Medicine, January 1993, found that one third of those interviewed used an unconventional medical approach within the last year. Unconventional therapies were defined in the study as "medical interventions not taught widely at U.S. medical schools or generally available at U.S. hospitals. Examples include acupuncture, chiropractic and massage therapy."[4]

One third of the subjects in the Harvard study using unconventional therapy visited a alternative practitioner an average of 19 times annually, paying an average of $27 per visit out of their own pocket. Those figures generalized to the U.S. population estimated that in one year Americans made 425 million visits to providers offering unconventional care and spent an estimated $10.3 billion, not covered by insurance. These numbers compare to 388 million visits to primary care physicians annually, and $12.8 billion spent out of pocket for all yearly hospitalizations. The majority of unconventional care was sought for chronic conditions that were being treated simultaneously by physicians – 70% of those patients did not inform their M.D.'s of their other therapy. This study indicates that conventional treatments are not answering the needs of many people. These Americans know there are other fruitful possibilities.

Conclusion: Good news

Modern science is beginning to understand and accept the relationship between our minds and our bodies. This relationship is an intuitive fact for many of us. The combination of intuition and science will provide a new approach to health and recovery. Endocrinologist Dr. Deepak Chopra says that,

"We are not physical machines that have learned how to think; we are consciousness, and the body is a print-out of our thoughts, feelings, interpretations and ideas."[5] Current scientific research proves the lack of separation between what we think of as our minds and our bodies. For example, the study of neuropeptides, messengers of the nervous system, has observed the biochemical interaction of emotion throughout the body, thereby demonstrating that mind and body are inseparable.[6] This fact has always lived in the language and the hearts of our poets, philosophers and mystics. This book encourages you to find inspiration in the new science that enhances the old wisdom.

Moving Back Into Your Body

There's no place like home.

– Dorothy
The Wizard of Oz

MODERN MEDICAL TREATMENT HAS A TEN-DENCY to inspire the "get me outta here!" response in patients. When we can't physically leave, we may remove ourselves mentally from the stressful situation. This self-protective reflex may have its place, but not in the day to day maintenance of health. We must appreciate the power of this interruption of our mind-body integration, and how it can occur, to understand the scope of balance that we need to thrive.

Scared out of our skin

Having surgery or being injured is a frightening and invasive experience. It is like a personal earthquake, with the disorientation, displacement, loss of privacy and control that are all side-effects of modern medical treatment. Before treatment, we must submit to interviews and examinations by strangers. If we are in a teaching hospital, we may be taught over, as if we are an inanimate educational tool.

Along the way, we may be humiliated and patronized by friendly faces who tell us we must expose ourselves for an examination or procedure, sometimes of questionable value. For example, when I was 13 years old, my sparse pubic hair was shaved in preparation for hip surgery. Why? Because it was once thought that shaving was hygienic. Shaving is no longer considered necessary, which leads one to wonder what other outmoded and insensitive habits are in place within the bureaucracy of medicine.

In a recent PBS documentary, Medicine at the Crossroads, a disturbing sequence showed an quadriplegic woman mouthing the words, "I am short of breath," over and over as the instructing physician discussed her case with interns. When the doctor finally noticed her attempts to communicate, he glanced at the wall of monitors attached to her, told her she was fine and breezed out of the room. Increased technology and mechanization of medicine has pulled doctors away from their own humanity and intuition. The poignant human experience of the paralyzed woman was utterly neglected.

These routine "little" surrenders and defeats drain away our sense of control. We tune out and ignore, or try to rise above and not care about the demoralizing nature of hospitalization. Our spirit relinquishes its temple in the name of modern medicine. At worst, we may be literally scared out of our skins. The withdrawal of consciousness may be so extreme that it resembles the out-of-body experiences described by those who have had near-death experiences. In these cases people report observing their bodies from a distance, as if watching a movie.

One cause of this withdrawal from the body can be a reaction to the drugs used for anesthesia, according to Dr. David Cheek, obstetrician for over 50 years, and pioneer in the medical uses of hypnosis. Cheek emphasizes research findings of state-dependent learning: That our bodies imprint every detail of a traumatic experience, as a survival mechanism, a warning system to protect us from future threats. The drugs used in surgical procedures, therefore, become associated with the trauma of that medical intervention by the body. When the drug is used again, the body "remembers" the past experience and can react badly if the experience was not positive. Dr. Cheek has found through his practice with hundreds of patients that traumatic birth experiences, in which the mother was anesthetized, can be remembered by the baby's body. The traumatic body memory can be reactivated many years later when the "baby" undergoes surgery. He feels that this phenomenon explains many unexpected negative reactions to anesthesia.[1]

While I was studying with Dr. Cheek, he suggested hypnosis to discover if I was being affected unconsciously by any of my four surgeries. While under hypnosis, I reported leaving my body during the surgery when I was ten years old. He regressed my mind to my birth. I reported that my mother's heavy sedation had affected me so severely that I felt dead and had to be revived. When I was exposed to anesthesia again, ten years later, my heart stopped. I reported looking for my parents to comfort me. I described being revived in such accurate detail, yet in a child's language, that Cheek believed it must have been a real occurrence. That surgery, which was originally scheduled for two hours, took over five hours. I became very ill after surgery. Ultimately my hip joint fused from disease.

My most successful surgery was also reviewed under hypnosis. I reported that before that operation the surgeon carefully explained what he was planning to do and that I would be responsible for the serious work of rehabilitation following the surgery. This discussion inspired my unconscious mind to stay present and alert during the surgery. I reported not leaving my body. I had an excellent recovery and enjoy a marvelous long-term outcome from that experience. Dr. Cheek felt so strongly about the importance of my case that he devoted several pages to it in his 1993 book, <u>Hypnosis: The Application of Ideomotor Techniques</u>. Given what science is finding out about the mind-body links, and in light of my personal experience, it seems clear that "evacuations" of the body during surgery can have serious physical and emotional consequences. Conversely, engaging the consciousness can have beneficial results.

Coming home

As you begin your journey toward balance, you must recognize that your body has a very emotional nature. With that realization, it is clear that you must be patient with your body, just as you would be with a child. Increasing your awareness, your self-knowledge, is a powerful tool for maintaining health, comfort, and the quality of life. It is the essential process of putting the driver (your awareness) back into the car (your body). Expanded awareness is best achieved when you have a genuine desire to learn, an equal willingness to take responsibility for your body, and a creative sense of discovery. To reap the rewards you seek, a methodical and gentle approach is essential.

As you know, many children do not get gentle treatment. This is where the mind-body split begins. They are taught to be tough, to "grow up." There is little sympathy for softness. Delicacy and sensitivity are considered weak. This attitude is usually communicated by parents who were treated harshly themselves as children. I am not talking about the horror of physical abuse, I am referring to the common undercurrent of hurried roughness by parents who are not aware of their effect on the child. Anatomy professor Ashley Montagu, in his classic, <u>Touching – The Human Significance of the Skin</u>, strongly states the problem:

> *The contemporary American family constitutes only too often an institution for the systematic production of mental illness in each of its members, as a consequence of its concentration on making each of them a "success"...entailing the suppression of emotion, the denial of love and friendship, while conveying an unvarying appearance of rectitude.(pg. 287)*

To remedy this, Montaqu recommends,

> *".....that in cultures of the Western world, and the United States particularly, parents express their affection for each other and for their children more demonstratively than they have in the past. It is not words so much as acts of affection and involvement that children, and, indeed, adults, require. (pg. 292)*

Touch is the child's first experience with the world. Research dating back to World War II by psychoanalysts John

Bolby and René Spitz observed that orphaned infants failed to develop normally without tender physical contact. Recent research with premature babies found that gentle massage increased their weight gain by 47%, when compared to the babies left alone in their incubators.[2] Gentleness does not equal weakness, it equals attentive care. Just as a flexible reed will spring back in the currents of a river, a gentle approach builds the awareness and confidence that supports personal resilience.

The following stories illustrate the benefits of being gentle with yourself.

When one of my clients was troubled with foot pain, I suggested that she take time to observe herself whenever she felt discomfort. Marilyn's first discovery was that the pain in her foot seemed to be related to the way she had been favoring her arthritic hip. Previously, I suggested that she use a tennis ball to gently massage the sole of her foot. As she used the ball to relieve the tension in her foot, she found a spot that made her feel sadness and fear. She allowed herself quiet time to feel her feelings. Marilyn realized that her emotions were a reaction to her upcoming hip surgery. Her body was calling attention to the sadness and fear she had been trying to ignore. When Marilyn acknowledged this, her physical pain disappeared. She was able to address and accept her emotional reaction to the surgery. This relief would not have been possible if she had taken a harsh, judgmental approach toward her body. One of the great secrets of the bodymind is that if we will just admit to our true feelings, simply take time to quietly listen to ourselves, often our pain will subside or become less troublesome.

Our feelings, like children, need our attention....and if we don't listen they will keep bothering us until we do pay attention! For example:

Anna came to me after a podiatrist recommended surgery for a stiffening toe joint. Her hope was to avoid the operation. She had been suffering for over a year with recurrent stress fractures in a metatarsal bone and general foot discomfort. Orthodics (special shoe inserts) had been prescribed a few years earlier and she had been wearing them regularly. In preparation for our first session, I suggested that she spend some time holding the toe that was bothering her and be aware of any thoughts or feelings that came up in relation to her feet. I also suggested she get her x-rays, so that we could study the injury.

When I arrived for our session she could hardly wait to tell me her discoveries. She traced her foot trouble back to a time when she worked at a very stifling job. She had forced her feet into uncomfortable, dressy shoes, which were a perfect metaphor for the whole situation. As she explored her history, she realized that the metatarsal fractures started after she began wearing the orthodics. She excitedly showed me the x-rays and how the orthodic design actually threw her foot off balance. This created an over correction that put pressure on her metatarsal bone, which could only break under the stress. She then tied the whole story together with insights about her deference to her doctors, former husband, and business partner. She felt that her feet were expressing a significant pattern in her life, breaking under the pressure to conform to male authority figures. I was very impressed at how much she had gotten from my simple suggestion to pay attention to her toe! Over the months that we worked together her discomfort disappeared, her posture improved and she was able to run pain-free. She also gained a renewed sense of direction in her life and clarity in her relationships.

In Marilyn's case it could be said, metaphorically, that she "could not stand" the thought of surgery. Anna was tired of having her "toes stepped on" and "walking on egg shells," so as not to disturb those she perceived to be in control. Each woman's foot pain was a body metaphor calling her to be more aware of her feelings and needs. Patience and awareness allowed each to get out of her intellect and appreciate how important her body was to her experience of life.

Conclusion

Moving back into your body mentally and emotionally after surgery or trauma is critical for complete healing. "Re-inhabiting" yourself requires increasing your bodymind awareness. This concept is the cornerstone of this book. You will find many ways of approaching this theme as you read. An attitude of true self-care is essential to developing self-awareness without judgment. In the next chapter I will discuss this crucial element to healing: love and acceptance.

Chapter 3

Love and Acceptance

*Out beyond ideas of right-doing and
wrong-doing there is a field,*

I'll meet you there.

– Rumi

L EARNING SELF-LOVE AND ACCEPTANCE IS ONE OF
life's greatest challenges. As we grow up, we invent and absorb a wide variety of "shoulds" about all
aspects of our lives. This is especially true for our bodies. Most of us feel our body should look a certain
way. We expect it to function perfectly and always be
there to support us. All our parts should last forever,
regardless of genetics or wear. So, when our body
starts to hurt or develops a problem that requires sur-

gery, and perhaps replacement, it can shake our basic foundations. Often we reject or isolate the "problem," the way a difficult child may be pushed aside in a family.

Our emotional attitudes play a large part in keeping us unaware and separate from our bodies. When we have endured pain and inconvenience, who wants to embrace the "trouble maker?!" One of my clients commented that she "hated" her arthritic hip. This is not an uncommon, nor mysterious reaction. It is, however, a damaging reaction because when we reject part of our body, we reject ourselves. Physiological disturbances can also contribute to our sense of alienation from troubled parts, which will be discussed in the next chapter. Establishing a positive relationship with yourself – all parts of you – holds rich rewards.

Coping with damage to our physical self

It is startling to face the fact that our body is imperfect or unable to retain its youthful resilience. It can be disturbing when our body doesn't work in its reliable, familiar ways. We may avoid admitting that our body will force us to compromise. Often we choose to turn away from ourselves in anger and fear, rather than face our situation constructively.

A very common reaction to injury or disability is to deny it. Our reasons for denial are very human. Pain and its implications can be frightening. We may be angry about recurring inconvenience. We don't want to make adjustments in our lifestyle. Perhaps we have had bad experiences with doctors in the past and therefore wish to avoid treatment at all costs. Maybe we just don't want to believe that we are vulnerable.

The world we live in encourages us to "gut it out," to "run through the pain." A symptom is considered weakness. Facing the truth that our body needs help can be very threatening to the ideal that we can control everything in our lives if we just work hard enough at it. This model of grinding perseverance has its roots in America's Puritan founders, who believed that sloth was the deadliest sin. This harsh approach to life is etched in our national psyche. It has suppressed our ability to care for ourselves by casting a shadow over the natural adjustment process we must go through following physical trauma.

Adjusting to change

A post-surgical nurse told me about a patient who told her wistfully, "I like my new knee....but, my old one...well, we had some good times..."When you have a severe injury, or a body part that needs to be replaced, there are at least three major sources of distress:

1. The loss of that part of your body as it has been known. Even if the part is diseased and has caused problems, it is part of yourself. It is familiar, known, natural: "Me."

2. Change of your posture, gestures or movement identity: the way you move through life, your physical expressiveness and your kinesthetic relationship with the world.

3. In the case of surgical implant, acceptance that there is now an artificial object in your body. Tissue from another or something inorganic....metal or plastic.... inanimate...a part...apart: "Not Me."

How do you face these facts? Some people don't think about it, but does that work? Is there subconscious rejection or isolation of your body occurring that will show up later in the need for further medical intervention? Possibly. Some people have conscious feelings of ambivalence or even hostility about a "foreign object" in their body. How does mental rejection of a "defective," or new part affect the immune response, body-image and movement patterns? I believe that such rejection can lead to difficulties.

Every day I see people sitting and moving in awkward ways that will eventually lead to damaging stress on their bodies. These patterns come from lack of awareness, avoidance of pain or compensation for weaknesses that have not been addressed. My first big insight about this came when I was in a ladies locker room. I happened to notice a woman's foot held in a tense and clumsy position, almost exactly like the position I used before I began working consciously to improve my movement patterns. When I glanced up from her foot to her hip, I saw that she had a scar just like mine!

The odd foot use is an attempt to stabilize a leg that is being used like a stick, instead of a flexible, living part of the body (based on my own and my clients' experience). In this physical pattern of denial, the hip is held still to avoid past pain and instability. It is a self-protective habit. Unfortunately, healthy function also gets interrupted. Circulation is reduced and mobility is restricted. Potentially difficult or challenging awareness is avoided, but so is the opportunity for optimal recovery. It is important to identify and correct those patterns which are no longer relevant

At a more delicate level, our immune system protects our body from what it perceives to be intruders or abnormal situations. Included in the functioning of the immune system are the brain, the spleen, the thymus gland, the bone marrow and the lymph nodes. With this complex network of organs and systems, the immune system can be affected by practically everything: biochemical changes, toxicity, hormones, behavior, emotions, diet or a combination of all of these factors. Norman Cousins says, "The immune system is a mirror of life, responding to its joy and anguish, its exuberance and boredom, its laughter and tears, its excitement and depression, its problems and prospects."[3] Studies in the growing field of psychoneuroimmunology document the ability of mood and emotion to affect the immune system positively and negatively. Therefore, it is beneficial for recovering patients to be in positive mental states. It follows that one's attitude toward a surgical implant would support or inhibit healing.

An example of the negative affects of attitude is the case of a young woman who had an unsuccessful hip replacement during her teens. She told me that after that surgery she had focused her adolescent conflicts on her hip, blaming it for her problems. She was very angry and rejecting of that part of her body. The procedure never stabilized properly. She felt that she consciously participated in her body's rejection of the prosthesis through her emotional rejection. Ultimately, her replacement had to be redone. Following her second surgery she tried to remove herself from the recovery experience through heavy use of marijuana, denying the importance of rehabilitation, literally "spacing out." There was a sense of shame as she talked about her hip. Today her outcome is still not satisfactory and will require more surgery.

Self-Care: The seed of recovery

It is nearly impossible to use your body well and treat it wisely when you feel hostile, fearful or harshly demanding toward some part of yourself. When I first began to pay attention to my body-image, I became aware of mentally amputating my operated leg, because it had caused me so much pain and difficulty. I also discovered an irrational fear that my leg might somehow fall off. Profound appreciation for the effects of my attitude came in my early twenties and marked the beginning of my true recovery:

My massage therapist gave me a homework assignment to "love" my operated hip every day for twenty minutes. Ever the conscientious student, I bought some massage oil and sat down to the task that very evening. Little did I know that what I would really need was courage and patience.

The first time I tried to lovingly massage my hip all I could do was angrily poke. The next day I held my hip gently, but soon impatience and annoyance set in and I stopped abruptly. The third day I tried again and felt fear welling up inside of me. I quit immediately. Fear came up again on the fourth day and again I retreated. On the fifth day when the fear came up like a tidal wave, I thought to myself, "this can't *kill* me, I might as well stay and face it." I kept gentle and firm physical contact with my leg and allowed the fear to wash through me.

My leg began to tremble violently. It quivered for what seemed like a long time. It never hurt. When I came to rest I felt calm. I sensed the distinct quality of ether (the anesthesia used in my childhood) in my stomach, reminiscent of post-surgical times past. A quarter-sized lump in my thigh between my scars was gone.(Had the drug been trapped in my body?) I also felt a new glimmer of peace within. The peace that love offers.

Love is essential for happiness in life. Love of self, love of life, love of others. Love of self is a simple phrase, however, it is the opposite of what we are taught. One is considered selfish, conceited, at best, self-indulgent if you love yourself. Still, to thrive, love is "the indispensable crowning grace."[1] The kind of loved that forges and maintains a strong, enduring partnership is the kind of love needed for yourself throughout ongoing recovery. This love is awake, loyal, patient and encouraging, it is brave in the face of uncertainty and pain. "To love means to stay when every cell says 'run!'."[2] It is the stuff of real nurturing and support for yourself. Optimal recovery, and life itself, requires this kind of compassionate commitment.

To accept the prosthesis, we must first compassionately accept our imperfection and vulnerability. Initially, I thought it was strange to have a big piece of metal screwed into my pelvis. Could it fall out? How did it affect my other tissues? Would I set off the metal detector in the airport again? Why did I have to be so different?!

Many years after my partial hip replacement, I became aware of how I unwittingly addressed this question of acceptance. Foremost in my mind at the time was that the surgery was my last chance. I made the conscious/unconscious decision that after several other failures, this one had to work. Years later I was more aware of what I had done in my mind: *I saw the metal cup in my pelvis as my own.* It had become *part of me,* completely engulfed, embraced, integrated by my bodily tissues. It is held in place by much more than the surgeon's screws. In my mental/emotional body image it is as normal as my other hip – normal for me – part of the unique individual that I am. We each have our "specialness;" that "cup" is part of mine.

While visiting a friend who had the aortic valve in his heart replaced with a valve from a pig, I observed that he spoke about the new valve as if it was completely separate from himself. It almost sounded as if the operation had happened to another person. I feel very strongly that one must really accept the "new part" for a long and happy recovery, so I asked John if he had given any thought to making the valve his own. The thought hadn't occurred to him. I talked about seeing his body carefully taking the new valve in, bathing it in his blood, welcoming it.

The next time I saw him, he commented on how useful that imagery had been to him. It created a subtle, but important shift. He talked about how easy it was for him to enjoy the idea of the new valve because it came from a pig, an animal for which he had always had a particular fondness. John, who at 59 ran his 50th marathon to mark the 6-month anniversary of his operation, was also delighted to learn that donor pigs are the racing pigs seen at fairs galloping for cookies and ice cream – one of his favorite treats.

~ ~

It is to our advantage to truly in-corporate – unite with thoroughly – these gifts of modern science; the new heart valve from a pig, a metal and plastic ball and socket for our hip, the organ of another. This is where modern medicine truly shines. And, here is where we have a clear opportunity to use our hearts and minds to facilitate our health. My experience is that the purposeful and positive incorporation of prosthesis enhances recovery.

Sometimes we resist accepting "good" things as much as we resist accepting "bad" things. If we have experienced difficulty in the past we don't want to get our hopes up, only to be disappointed. Our doctors may discourage optimism, perhaps thinking it will encourage risk-taking. This is where we must take the chance of believing in ourselves, in the inner strength that has brought us thus far. Keep looking until you find something or someone who you feel you can trust to offer logical and responsible possibilities to help you. Openness, balanced with necessary caution, can yield unexpected and fruitful options.

Trust: Surrendering control

Love and acceptance call on us to surrender, to trust in what we cannot see or completely understand: They call upon us to have faith. A client recovering from her seventh surgery articulated that fact when I asked her to contrast her approach to her recent and unexpectedly successful hip surgery with her earlier hip surgery, which was marred by bone erosion, migration of the prosthesis and chronic pain. She told a remarkable story of personal realization. It is an inspiring example of how the shift from a brittle and illusory stance of being "in control" to a position of acceptance and responsiveness can transform the rehabilitation experience.

Judith's string of surgeries began with a near-fatal car accident at the age of 17. Three of her friends died. She escaped with a crushed hip and other broken bones. Her family rallied around her, bolstering her with the image that she was a "survivor." However, she was never given the opportunity to grieve the loss of her friends, her hip, or the abrupt end to her youthful freedom.

After two years of medical treatment she was left with a fused hip. Her doctors and family were satisfied with her outcome. She forged ahead, marrying at the age of 19. Before long she was mother of four. At the age of 35 she had a total hip replacement to restore movement to her hip. Now a single mother, she moved her children to a new community so that she could go to college. She ultimately completed a graduate degree and became a psychotherapist.

At 45 she was forced to have the hip replacement partially revised. Following that surgery, her physical problems and her personal awakening began. Judith described herself at that time as a heavy smoker who paid little attention to her diet or alcohol intake, coping with the stress of her illness with "false will." Up until that time she had managed her life by willfully conquering everything in her path, lacking a perspective which gave a sense of the larger meaning or order in her life. She intellectually "controlled everything." She denied the deterioration of her hip condition. Serious complications following a hysterectomy forced her to change.

She became very ill after the difficult surgical procedure in which her intestines were punctured. A week after the surgery she was quite weakened, her family and doctors becoming very concerned. In desperation her daughter sought out a spiritual healer who offered a prayer to be read to Judith. This moment of prayer provided the turning point. Judith vividly described crying with relief and having the distinct feeling of "falling out of (her) place of false will and false self, into the arms of the Divine." Her recovery moved forward from that point. A year later, when she faced another hip replacement her approach was completely opposite to her former, "tough it out" attitude.

Judith has given great care to all aspects of her recovery from this surgery, which her surgeon considered a real long shot because of massive bone and muscle degeneration. There is a very open and humble quality to her demeanor as she carefully monitors her emotional, spiritual and physical states. Reflection and meditation have become cornerstones in her life. She refers to her "healing hip," rather than referring to her "bad hip" which I hear so many other clients say. As a post-menopausal woman, she has – remarkably – generated significant bone growth with the help of twice weekly electro-acupuncture and weekly sessions with me, including education, bone-tracing bodywork and visualization. One of the first things I did was give her a real femur (thigh bone), one that was strong and whole, as a tool to make concrete the image of healthy bone she was creating in her meditation.

Witnessing Judith's progress has been an inspirational gift. Hers is a truly self-loving and reverential approach. She has applied the principles of deep self-awareness and care, transforming her former approach to life. When she described herself five years earlier I could hardly believe it, the contrast was so great. Today there is a quiet spirit of awareness and real self care surrounding her. I cannot imagine her smoking or abusing herself in any other way.

The profound beauty of her story is that she is recovering beyond her surgeon's wildest dreams. She found peace and order within herself that guides her to know and trust what her body needs. Shortly after surgery, her surgeon told her that her hip muscles resembled those of "a paraplegic" and to expect no significant improvement. She would always be very weak, in his opinion. He was also concerned with the thinness of her thigh bone. I strongly encouraged her to meditate on rinsing that, and any other discouraging comments, from her mind. At her six-month check-up he was surprised by the improvement in her muscle mass, and in a state of near disbelief over the fact that she had actually accomplished visible bone growth in areas that had been severely degenerated. I expect that she will continue to surprise him.

Conclusion

Injury or recovery from surgery calls upon us to see the difference between self-indulgence and necessary self-care, and find new skills within. Judith's story demonstrates the power of love and self-care. She transformed her previously impatient, unaware and unhealthy life. She said that the only time she did slow down previously was when she was sick. Now, she has given herself such a depth of attention and respect that she is recovering in a balanced way, unlike anything she has experienced before. Her story is a perfect bridge from love and acceptance, to the dynamics of self-support discussed in the next chapter.

Chapter 4

Supporting Yourself

Animate the earth within us:
We then feel the Wisdom underneath supporting all.

– Neil Douglas-Klotz
<u>Prayers of the Cosmos</u>

WHEN I LOOKED UP "SUPPORT" IN MY COM-
PUTER'S thesaurus, these words were listed:
livelihood, maintenance, sustenance, backing, pro-
motion, blessing, favor, succor, brace, foundation,
reasoning, bolster, strengthen, advance, advocate,
champion. The antonyms of support include opposi-
tion, weaken and neglect. These are all powerful
words when applied to health and rehabilitation. Will
we strengthen or weaken ourselves? Will we maintain
or neglect ourselves? Do we believe we can sustain

ourselves, or will we deny our abilities? Again, the concerns of health become the metaphoric questions about how we live our lives.

History of our support

To address the issue of self-support it is useful to step back and look at what we learned about support as a child. Did we learn to truly support ourselves from those around us or did we learn habits of neglect? Our modern society does not teach the importance of personal time for reflection and regeneration. In fact, self-neglect is the prevailing behavior, especially when you consider the type of deep attention needed for healing and renewal of the body and soul. Parents by definition fill their children's external needs. They must keep the household operating; there is little time for themselves. Thus, they rarely can model self-care skills to their children. Instead, models of overwork and martyrdom are the norm. Children learn that it is most noble to support others at the expense of themselves, because they see no other alternative.

My early childhood was typical of this conventional model of self-support. I was the first of 4 children. My younger twin sisters also had congenital hip dislocations which required several surgeries. My mother's hands were more than full. My father was an absent, overextended clinical social worker and university professor. Since I was bright and independent, I'm sure they assumed that I was capable of "taking care of myself." I felt well cared for and loved. Yet, when my hip began hurting after the birth of my brother and a move to a new community (which I did not like), not one adult stopped to explore my emotional state. It was assumed that my long dormant hip problem was the culprit. The x-rays supported that idea. So, I was scheduled for surgery.

I was given "the best" medical care, yet was that support? With hindsight, I say no. I learned after many years of self-observation that my hip begins to trouble me when I feel overwhelmed or abandoned (unsupported). Now when I notice a bit of achiness I take time to be compassionate with myself. I examine ways to take better care of myself in my relationships or other life situations. I do physical self-care practices which help me relax and feel more balanced in my body. Often just a warm, candle lit bath and a quiet evening can avert further discomfort. My clients report that my suggestions to slow down and care for themselves help them avoid pain and the fear that comes with it. As we saw with Marilyn in the first chapter, discomfort may only be a plea from inside to take time to listen. Over and over in my private sessions when I encourage clients not to resist their pain, but just to observe it, they report that the discomfort melts away within a few minutes.

When I was a 10 year old, with a new brother, new home, new school, new town, it is easy to see why I would have felt overwhelmed and alone. The shallowness of my hip socket was real, but was it bad enough to necessitate immediate surgery? (Research finds emotional not physical problems cause most low back pain.) An approach that included care for my emotional life might have put off surgery. Most certainly, emotional support would have positively affected my recovery. As it happened, without understanding my emotional state, the surgery was followed by serious complications. Research has found that patients with more stress may have more post surgical complications.[1] Addressing my adjustment problems and checking for negative subconscious influences through hypnosis, as discussed in Chapter One, could have reduced my stress level, reduced my pain, and prepared me for a better surgical outcome.

Learning self support

The severity of my complications created a new level of awareness within my family. My father searched all over the country for the best surgeon to help me. Ultimately, I was sent from my home in San Francisco to Boston. The surgeon in Boston required an extensive rehabilitation program. My mother worked with me twice a day on my exercises, in addition to taking me swimming. We talked about how the movements would create smooth joint surfaces, unconsciously activating my mind's participation through imagery. She was a dedicated partner in my recovery, and taught me great lessons about love and commitment. That experience instilled in me the conviction that I could affect my rehabilitation; I could support my recovery and myself in patient, loving and practical ways. Her care gave me a priceless gift.

Active awareness

Essential to self-support is heeding the communication from your physical self. Learning to observe your body and how to direct your awareness are powerful tools that you can use to create new solutions to old problems. At the University of Massachusetts, Dr. Jon Kabat-Zinn uses mindfulness meditation techniques to help chronic pain patients cope with and reduce their symptoms.[2] In this program, similar to my approach, people learn to simply observe their pain without judgment. Since its founding in the early 1980's, Dr. Kabat-

Zinn's program has helped hundreds of patients who were not cured by conventional medical therapies by calling on their bodies inner resources. Throughout this discussion, keep in mind that each area of support; attitudinal, biochemical, neurological, and structural interacts with and is influenced by the others in a dance that is yet to be fully understood.

Our biochemical support

Science proves that directing our awareness influences body processes. Biofeedback illustrates these findings quite clearly. Using sophisticated monitoring equipment, biofeedback tracks how attention to a specific area of the body affects circulation, by temperature and other changes. Circulation is the basis of healthy tissues, organs, joints, and metabolism, because blood carries nourishment, oxygen, and informational substances (the messengers of the nervous, endocrine and immune systems) throughout the body. Circulation also carries away tissue wastes. These processes are essential to complete healing after surgery.

A breakthrough area of research, psychoneuroimmunology, (the study of how the mind, nervous and immune systems interact) has discovered bridges between the systems in our bodies once considered separate by science. The nervous system, long thought of as wiring to the brain, turns out to be a complex network of electrical and biochemical relationships interacting with cells of the endocrine and immune systems. Certain white blood cells throughout the body are equipped with the molecular equivalent of antennae tuned specifically to receive messages from the brain. These cells have been referred to as "bits of the brain floating around in the body."[3] This field of science is very new; however, researchers are hopeful to someday define the processes of thought and emotion as they spring from the intricate physiology of the body-mind.

Our neurological support

The brain is encoded with a model of our body that is constantly modified by input from the peripheral nerves of our limbs and skin. It follows that this model can be used for recovery. Consciously activating this inner "blueprint" through the intellect, imagery, sensory awareness and movement can help the body function, fully integrated.

Research in neurology and neuropsychology is beginning to uncover how injury to the body affects the encoding in the brain. Experiments immobilizing monkeys' fingers show that the coding in the brain disappears for the stilled finger. Areas of the brain representing the hand surrounding the restricted finger enlarge and fill in the area of the brain where the "lost" digit was represented. The unmoving finger literally loses its place in the brain.[4]

Oliver Sacks, M.D., in his rich personal report of severe leg injury, A Leg to Stand On, describes absolute alienation from his leg that was gravely injured, then immobilized in a cast. Sacks describes the experience of loss found in the above mentioned research, years before those experiments were conducted:

> *I turned at once to my leg(in the cast), with a keen, startled and almost fierce attention...It was utterly*

strange, not-mine, unfamiliar...It was absolutely not-me – and yet, impossibly, it was attached to me – and even more impossibly, "continuous" with me...In particular, it no longer seemed like a "home."...It didn't "go" anywhere. It had no place in the world." (pp. 72–73)...For what was disconnected was not merely nerve and muscle, but as a consequence of this, the natural and innate unity of body and mind. The "will" was unstrung as precisely as the nerve muscle. The spirit was ruptured as precisely as the body. (pp. 96)

The brain modifies itself rapidly and is dependent upon the body's mobility and use for its own organization. (In a later injury, Sacks felt the same sense of loss of his dislocated shoulder after only two hours of immobilization in a cast.) This understanding of brain-body interaction has important implications for recovery from trauma and surgery. Movement is essential for the return of function and personal orientation. Sacks describes his experience after standing and taking his first steps in a walking cast. Accomplishing these first steps required the spontaneously return of the deepest music of the body, like a physical Aha!

A miracle seemed to have happened. The reality of my leg, the power to stand and walk again, had been given to me, descended upon me like grace. Now, reunited with my leg – with the part of myself that had been excommunicated, in Limbo – I found myself full of tender regard for it, and stroked the cast. I felt an immense feeling of Welcome for the leg lost, now returned. The leg had come home, to its home, to me. In action the body had been broken, and only now,

with the return of bodily action as a whole, did the
body itself feel whole again. (ibid. pp. 110)

Patients are encouraged to get up and move soon after surgery. However, I hear of people who move very little after coming home from the hospital. These reports come to me from clients who are surprised by how poorly an inactive acquaintance is recovering. Consistently, my clients who are active and aware of their bodies fare better than those who are not. Now we can understand why: the brain literally "forgets" how to move the affected limb. Movement helps the brain and body re-collect.

Much of what I do with clients is retraining their movement patterns through intellectual and physical understanding of how to walk, for example. It is useful to practice with the healthier side that still has the body-brain wiring intact. The weaker side can literally learn from its stronger counterpart. Imagining the movement of the affected limb also prepares it for regaining coordination. This concept is a basic element of the Feldenkrais Method.[5] Explorations in general sensory awareness, presented in Chapter Seven, are equally important. I have observed that intellectual and intuitive understanding enhances the ability to move when the motor coordination is still in the state of memory loss. The principles of love, acceptance and support solidify the return of normal body-image.

Neurological responses and improved motor functioning have been documented using biofeedback technology. Dr. Bernard Brucker at the University of Miami School of Medicine uses biofeedback techniques to help people disabled by brain and spinal cord damage.[6] Brucker's Biofeedback Laboratory at the Department of Orthopedics and Rehabilitation teaches patients to use their existing neural cells in the brain and spinal cord to regain muscle control. This procedure depends on sensitive computer equipment to monitor neural activity. Patients are able to develop and expand physical control by watching the changes in their bodies monitored on computer screens. This visual observation replaces the natural sensations and reflex feedback that have been lost through injury or disease. It appears that patients activate new neuropathways, which gives them greater use of their bodies.

Another example of this is the fact that we increase our number of active brain cells when we learn new things. Landmark research at the University of California at Berkeley found that rats raised in "enriched environments" (with lots of toys) had brains significantly larger than the rats raised in barren cages. All the rats started out with equivalent brains, but challenging activities expanded what was naturally present.[7] We can do the same thing, anytime, with our brains and peripheral nervous systems.

A client of mine learned biofeedback several years before coming to me. She described it as a way of getting past the self-doubt that had previously undermined her ability to help herself. By watching the monitors track the changes in her body, she learned to make random improvement become voluntary, within her control. She observed that when she put too much effort into it, the improvement disappeared. Developing a sense of trust in her body's "knowing" how to find balance when she gave herself quiet attention was her most valuable and sustaining lesson. She likened her experience of my hands-on work and self-care assignments to her biofeedback experience, each providing new tools in developing her sense of conscious participation in her recovery from surgery.

Our structural support

To understand your physical support system you must begin with your skeleton. As an experiment, stop for a moment, close your eyes and turn your attention to your bones, by-passing your muscles and other soft tissues. What do you feel? How do you feel? Do you feel anything!? Few of us have an active sense of our skeleton. The idea of feeling my bones was completely alien to me the first time I tried it. But those bones have got to be in there – what else could be holding us up?

Developing awareness of my bones has been very practical. Due to surgical nerve damage, I have reduced sensation on the outer part of my thigh above my knee. That knee is unstable, tending to buckle inward. At the suggestion of a teacher, I began to focus my attention on the outer knob (condyle) of my thigh bone, which is the numb area. When I did this my knee was more stable and my pattern of walking improved. This is another example of the brain expanding neuropathways to increase function, as demonstrated in biofeedback research. I observed gradual improvement as I incorporated this numb and previously unconscious area into my body awareness. My expanded awareness helped me maintain and continue the improvement.

Our skeleton is a wonderful structure, naturally designed to support us effortlessly. Each bone is contoured to facilitate the function it serves. A small shift in posture or placement can make a big difference in comfort. A few basic anatomy points will help to explain this. We will move from the ground up to appreciate how each part supports the next. It is important to understand your joints and keep them all as

flexible as possible. Chapter Seven will provide several ways
to increase and maintain your flexibility.

The feet and ankles

The feet are the foundation for all other aspects of your support. Many people walk on only part of their feet, often getting little balance from their heel, which has a direct
relationship to the stability of the ankle, knee and hip joints.
Attention to the feet is often the single most useful tool for
correcting walking problems and discomfort, my clients have
found. The key is to think of the four weight bearing points
of each foot, and balance your weight between them. (Figure
4.1) Developing a sense of the width of your heel is especially

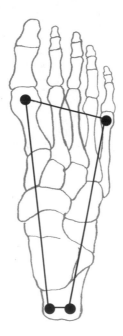

Figure 4.1 Four Weight-Bearing Points of the Foot.

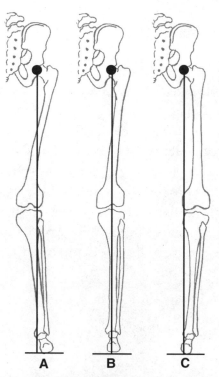

Figure 4.2 Foot/Ankle Relationship - view of right leg from behind in three positions: A) ankle collapsing inward(pronation) B) balanced alignment C) ankle collapsing outward(supination).

important. People often walk as if their heel is narrow, like a high heeled shoe. This makes it easy for the ankle to collapse inward or outward. The illustration (Figure 4.2) shows the result of this "pronation" or "supination". It is possible to learn to be conscious of how your foot meets the ground and control the balance of the heel and ankle, rather than becoming dependent upon artificial support.

The knees

I have observed that the knees can become uncomfortable and/or hypermobile when the range of movement is reduced in the hips, ankles or feet. When the knees move in ways they are not designed to move, problems can arise.

The surfaces of the knee joint are big and there is a system of strong connective tissue to stabilize the joint. The tibia (the bone we call our shin) is a dense weight-bearing shaft with a head that creates a broad platform for the femur (bone of the thigh) to rest into.(Figure 4.3) Proper alignment of the shaft and platform of the tibia facilitates healthy movement of the knee and supports the hip and upper body. The foundation of this alignment is the foot. Major circulatory pathways pass through the back of the knee. These pathways can be compressed if you lock or push your knees backward. It is beneficial to develop the habit of having a slight, soft bend in your knees to encourage good circulation.

The hips

It is essential to understand the true location of your hip joints to understand how they function. Many people are unclear about this most basic element of their support. First of all, the joints are very low and work like a hinge. To discover this in yourself, bend your knees slightly, keep your back

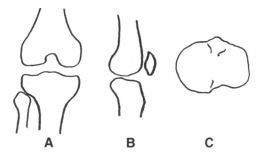

Figure 4.3 The Knee - A) front view of right knee without kneecap B) inner side view of right knee C) looking down on platform of tibia.

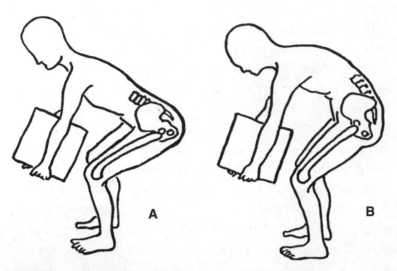

Figure 4.4 Location of Hip Joints – proper bending from hips(A) rather than lower back(B)

straight and lean forward letting your buttocks extend behind you. Put your fingers in the crease that is created in the front. Voila! You will find your hip joints. Bending from this hinge protects your lower back (Figure 4.4a). People often mistake the top of their pelvic bones for their hip joints, and therefore reverse the natural curve in the low back every time they sit or lean over, by bending too high. (Figure 4.4b)

My favorite fact about hip joints is that they are just as far apart as your ears. For a week after I learned this I kept taking off my sunglasses and comparing the width of the glasses to the location of my hip joints. The important element of that fact is to learn how central your support is from your hips. (Figure 4.5)

Many people, women in particular, think of their hips as being the widest part of their seat. That is where we take our hip measurements, after all. That area is actually the greater trochanter, which is part of the femur. It is a couple of inches lower and to the outside of the ball and socket joint. Assum-

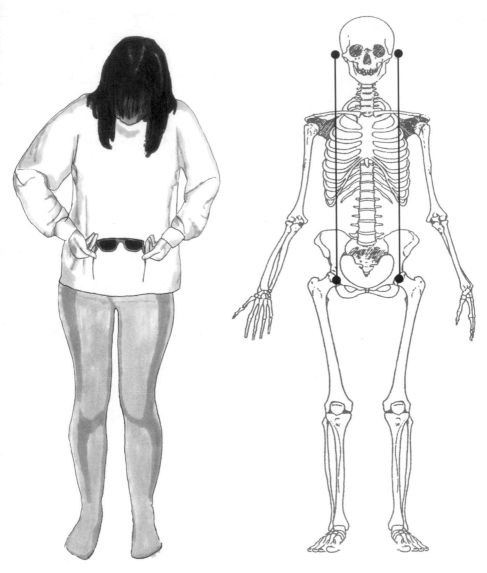

Figure 4.5 Central Position of Hip Joints

ing that your support comes from that trochanter area can feel precarious, causing you to shift from side to side when you walk (like the great femme fatales in spiked heels). Learning to feel the central nature of your support gives a feeling of balance and collectedness that transports energy up through the pelvis into the spine and makes walking easier and lighter overall.

The spine

A normal spine is made up 24 separate vertebrae plus the large wedge-shaped sacrum and tailbone at the base. Each vertebra is shaped differently, slightly wedged, to create the gentle, self-supporting S-curve of the spine when viewed from the side. (There are seven cervical, 12 thoracic, 5 lumbar, 5

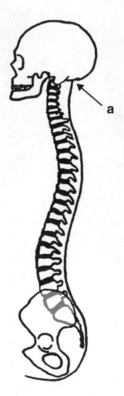

Figure 4.6 Profile of Spine. a) The Head and Neck Relationship.

fused sacral vertebrae and four coccygeal bones of the tail.) Many neck and back problems are created when the subtle natural curves are straightened, reversed or exaggerated by poor posture, imbalance of strength in the complementary muscle groups and inefficient movement habits. A healthy spine, free of tension, will support itself, leaving the muscles available to initiate movement. (Figure 4.6) A good head position enables you to have a feeling of natural ease and length in your spine.

The head

The balance point of the head, where it is supported by the neck, can be found easily by placing one finger on each side below your ear and directly behind your jaw bone. An inch or so in from where you are touching are the dished surfaces where your head rests on your "atlas", the top neck vertebra. Many people drop their head forward or back, as if their face outweighs the back of the head, or vice versa. These postural misunderstandings create a variety of strains that can transfer down through the whole body. In reality, the face and the back of the head naturally balance one another (the mass of the front and back being equal). It is easy to carry your head lightly when you remember that it is supported right in the center. The trick is to *continue* remembering that so that you break your old habits! This is an example of how increased self-awareness can serve you, helping you to make your life more comfortable. (Figure 4.6a)

The chest and arms

Your ribs, shoulders and arms are supported by good spinal alignment and head/neck relationship. When your spine is in its natural order, your ribs and sternum hang flexibly. There are movable joints where each rib meets the spine in the back and sternum in the front. These joints allow the expansion and release of your chest with each breath. Your shoulder blades ride on the back of your ribs, attached in the front to your collarbone. Your collarbone is jointed with your sternum. When your shoulders ride easily, your arm movement is unrestricted and your hands can be comfortable at their tasks. If you have trouble with hand or wrist discomfort observe how you use your shoulders, they may hold the key. (Figure 4.7) An easy and effective way to keep your upper body open and comfortable is presented in Chapter Seven.

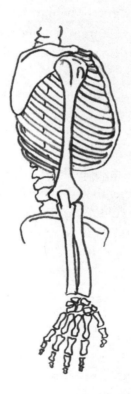

Figure 4.7 Chest, Shoulder and Arm Relationship

Conclusion

As you have observed, supporting yourself has many facets; from emotional sensitivity and persistence, to the subtle, bone-deep awareness that comes from feeling your inner architecture. Supporting yourself means developing trust in yourself, mind and body. Now, with the blessings of modern technology, we know we can observe, appreciate and influence the self-healing tools within us. Based on what has been discussed in the first three chapters, you know that it is possible to enhance your inner processes consciously. You can help yourself get better by activating new neuropathways and your body's other healing resources: the infinite circuit of mind supporting body supporting mind.

Next we will examine our greatest obstacle to healing: The Bermuda Triangle of pain, fear and depression.

Chapter 5

The Bermuda Triangle

…And only if we arrange our life in accordance with the principle which tells us that we must trust in the difficult, then what appears to us as the most alien will become our most intimate and trusted experience…

Perhaps everything that frightens us is, in its deepest essence, something helpless that wants our love.

– Rainier Maria Rilke

THE BERMUDA TRIANGLE IS A STRETCH OF SEA IN the North Atlantic legendary for the unexplained disappearances of ships and planes that cross into its borders. Like the Bermuda Triangle, the triple whammy of pain, fear and depression ambushes many an unsuspecting person, capsizing personal progress and happiness. These emotional tidal waves *can* be beneficial when understood as timely opportunities to grow and change. In this chapter we will examine the interlocking dynamics of the pain-fear-depression triangle and explore ways to use it constructively.

Physiology of pain, fear and depression

Have you ever noticed that your sense of yourself vanishes when you are caught in life's cross currents? You may look "fine" to others, but you feel lost, invisible, without moorings. This reactive emotional pattern is rooted in a basic survival mechanism: fear and its mask depression, in response to pain. This primitive survival pattern often undermines our best efforts in a complex modern world. The instinctual base of the brain overwhelms the more rational cerebral cortex and we get swamped by a wave of our own biochemical soup that may move us to react against our better judgment.

Understanding the body's complex psycho-physiological interactions has been one of the primary scientific challenges of this century. The sciences that study mind/body interactions are in the middle of a revolution. Hundreds of scientists are conducting research through programs created when Congress declared the 1990's the "Decade of the Brain." New medical technology, especially sophisticated computer imaging techniques, allow the observation of subtle body processes barely dreamed of a few years ago. Researchers can now observe how our nervous systems, immune systems, metabolic systems and mental states are highly interactive. Although conclusive evidence is years away in some areas, the potential for understanding what has been a mystery is tremendous. What follows is an introductory discussion of some of what is already known about mind/body interaction.

Pain

Pain is a basic sensory experience we humans share with all animal life. Its function is to warn us of actual or potential tissue damage. Physical pain is thought to be activated by neurotransmitters which are released whenever and wherever body tissue is injured. These chemicals in turn stimulate the pain receptors of the nervous system and trigger chemicals that initiate healing. Pain tells us to stop what we are doing to hurt ourselves. Without the information it provides we could do terrible damage to ourselves. Just imagine if you could not feel a hot stovetop or the edge of a kitchen knife. Pain's primary job is to protect us. Those who insist on ignoring their pain often cause serious problems for themselves.

Pain is a very personal thing. We all perceive the stimulus for pain at the same level (for example, heat is perceived as painful at 44–46 C), but our ability to tolerate the pain may be very different. Many cultural and psychological factors affect how pain is tolerated by an individual. A frequently cited example of this is how a seriously injured person may work to save others in an emergency, oblivious to his/her own pain.

The great variation in human experience of pain suggests that there are natural mechanisms that can modify the perception of pain. Medical research has found that we have natural opiates (beta-endorphins and enkephalins) that are released when we are in pain that lessen our awareness of pain. They are the body's natural response to the stress of pain. Hypnosis, natural child-birth methods, meditation and other successful methods of pain control are believed to tap into these natural pain-reducing mechanisms.

The ongoing discoveries of complex interactions in our psychobiology serve to underline the need to include emotional and intellectual variables in the maintenance of health and comfort. A new day will dawn, when science is able to understand the emotional origins of pain, such as the deep muscle contractions that cause "heartache," "a pain in the neck," and other afflictions we describe with body metaphors. Our physical and emotional experience may be explained, and, hopefully, *respected*, making way for simple and direct methods of treatment that care for the whole patient, body and soul. It is my belief that the body's response to fear will shed light on how those metaphors manifest.

Fear

One of humankind's basic instincts is to avoid pain, both physical and emotional. The body's "fight-or-flight" response musters the body's resources to fight or flee in the face of a *perceived* danger. When a threat triggers this response the senses sharpen and hormones flood the body, increasing heart rate and heightening muscle tension to meet the challenge. The lower brain prepares the body before the cerebral cortex (where thought occurs in humans) has had time to explain the threat. This hair-trigger system is lifesaving in situations where physical danger erupts. Unfortunately, this same system is activated in situations that are more emotionally than physically threatening. It is this survival response that underlies much of the stress of life today. Our body prepares to fight or flee, and in most cases we do neither. It is not uncommon for this heightened state of stress to become chronic, wearing on many body systems.

Conditioned Fear. Dr. Walter Cannon, the Harvard physiologist who first observed the fight-or-flight response in laboratory animals in the early 1900's, said that fear was defined as "the premonition of pain."[1] The body braces itself. The mind expects the present and future to be like the past. This reaction can be explained by what scientists refer to as "state-dependent learning." State-dependent learning, or conditioning, programs our physiology (and therefore our emotions) to "expect" a certain experience to follow another specific experience, based on past events. This kind of learning was referred to in Chapter Two regarding patients' adverse reactions to anesthesia because of earlier negative experiences. Similarly, laboratory rats can be conditioned to fear a bright light by exposing them to mild electrical shock simultaneously with the light. This is learning by association. Eventually exposure to the light will evoke fear without the shock. The fear is experienced, regardless of the present reality. It has been shown that these rats can unlearn this fear response through repeated experience of the light without the shock. This unlearning of the fear reaction takes place in the "thinking" part of the brain, the cortex.[2]

We, too, can unlearn our reactive habits. Fear is a reaction to conditions suspiciously like those that have caused us pain in the past. With awareness of our learned responses, we can choose consciously to see that the present situation is new, and therefore, can be different. We can also recognize that we are better equipped to handle the situation that is like the one that once caused us pain, physical and emotional. For example, I have worked with many people who were abused as children. As adults, they feel fearful and powerless in the face of authority. When they realize that their fears are based on their experience as children, a time when they truly were vulnerable and completely dependent on the authority figures around them, their present situation becomes more manageable. They learn to use their adult skills of communication and planning, allowing the childlike feelings of danger to recede.

Despite our alleged superiority to lab rats, it still takes any human many trials (or at least lots of talking to oneself) before we can see the new situation for what it is: NEW. This recognition allows for a fresh experience. In a stressful situation, staying in the present is aided by careful observation of the micro–seconds of sensory experience. Sometimes I have had to reassure myself moment by moment: "Yes, I'm okay now...and now...and now...still okay?... yes...and now..." I use this method on bumpy airplane rides to limit my gray hair production.

Accurate information always helps when any situation evokes fear. For example, learning something about air currents helped me feel more comfortable while flying in an airplane. Learning facts about anatomy and physiology reassured me and made me appreciate the wisdom and miraculous complexity of the body's systems of basic functioning and self-repair. Fear is clearly an important instinct; however, the dangers in our world are not as simple as they were when the human species began. We must remember to examine our fears and ask, "Must I really be afraid?"

Depression

Depression is one of the most widely discussed and written about afflictions of modern society. In a push to find lucrative pharmacological cures, drug companies have poured millions of dollars into research. Here the "mind-body problem" frustrates the hope for a simple solution. Much of the research has restricted itself to body OR mind, not attempting to account for the mind-body interaction, thus offering only partial explanations. It is nearly impossible to keep pace with the new theories and research findings. The following will introduce the basic thinking on the origins of depression which integrate psychological and biological components, followed by environmental and nutritional factors.

In his ambitious work, <u>Depression: A Psychobiological Synthesis</u>, Paul Willner reviews hundreds of research papers in order to find a balanced explanation for depression. His final analysis suggests that ongoing psychological stress may be responsible for many of the biological factors associated with depression. He concludes that four elements of life experience make one most vulnerable to developing depression:

1. Ongoing stress and strain – marital, financial or work related.

2. Lack of social support.

3. Loss of a parent in childhood.

4. An introverted and negative pattern of thought.

It is easy to see how any of these factors would stimulate a variety of fears, most significantly survival-based fears of loss of love, shelter or community. These fears trigger the metabolic fight-or-flight response. A constant state of alarm wears down the body's ability to stay in balance, literally overloading its own biochemical and neurological circuits. The body's natural reaction is to conserve energy and withdraw (the symptoms of depression), until the body and emotions can regain their balance. The neurochemical interactions of this process are not yet completely understood, yet the pattern is logical.[3]

Hormonal imbalances are important players in our moods. The underproduction of thyroid is a well known culprit. As any woman knows, imbalances of progesterone and estrogen are strong factors. Reduced exposure to sunlight is a factor in some cases. Melatonin a natural sedative hormone, is suppressed by daylight. Seasonal Affective Disorder (SAD), with symptoms of depression and lethargy, is brought on by the increased levels of melatonin during the shorter days in winter.

Finally, it turns out that the "sugar blues" are actually a hormonal response. Refined sugar is so similar to our naturally produced glucose that it escapes digestive processing, where the amounts of glucose are automatically balanced with oxygen by the body. When the glucose level rapidly rises, the brain registers the imbalance and stimulates the pancreas and adrenal glands (primary participant in the fight-or-flight response) to pour hormones directly into the blood. The result is the familiar "sugar high."

Depression hits when the blood sugar drops in a rebound effect. Low energy, nervousness and a clouded mind are all symptoms of the body's struggle to re-balance. These mental and physical extremes happen because sugar depletes many of the body's essential nutrients including protein, vitamin B, zinc, chromium and manganese, which are all necessary for mental and emotional functioning, and whose depletion has been associated with depression, fatigue and low blood sugar. In his book, <u>Staying Healthy with the Seasons</u>, Elson Haas, M.D., reports that when he "...kicked the 'sugar habit'.[he] experienced... the best, most consistent, and most productive energy I had ever known."(pg. 115)

For our own well-being, it is important to understand and work to alleviate depression. In any discussion of human functioning, individual differences in biology and experience must be recognized. Where one person is vulnerable, another may be innately strong. In each model presented above, the significant element is that stress is created in the body, and the natural reflex to withdraw and conserve energy becomes dominant. Awareness of the variables provides us with options for change.

Using awareness to break the cycle

Fear is a basic psychological challenge that we must face from birth. Fear forces us to test reality: Is our fear of something real or is the "danger" an illusion? Is the outcome which we dread unavoidable, or do we have the resources to prevail? Depression takes over when we abandon hope that we can make the changes necessary to avoid pain. To meet the challenge we must gather information, as much information as possible. Detailed understanding of our condition helps us to come back to ourselves with clarity. We can begin to see the possibilities for addressing our situation.

Investigate your pain

What is the pain? (Allow yourself to feel the sensation, without pushing it away.)

What is its origin, in the broadest sense?

What can you do about it?

Pain is information that *something* is not right. (Don't assume you know what.) Pain evokes fear. We are afraid the pain means something is terribly wrong. We are afraid the pain will never stop, and only grow worse. This reaction causes constriction in the body – the fight-or-flight response – usually aggravating the discomfort. Pain makes us feel out of control. Fear interrupts our ability to cope constructively with the sensation. To be constructive, we can accept pain as a tool for problem solving.

A methodical approach can be very fruitful. First recognize that the pain is not YOU. In the past you may have had chronic pain, weakness, limitations. With an open and curious mind you have the opportunity to shape your present and future experience. When a twinge of pain comes, notice it, but don't clutch the pain as evidence that you are sentenced to a life of suffering. Learn from it: Did I step awkwardly?... How can I move more efficiently?...Am I doing too much?...Is there something else in my life I am not listening to, so that the pain forces me to slow down, pay attention, get depressed?...Use the pain. Don't push it away (trying to push it away takes tremendous effort). Listen to it. Have compassion for yourself.

I learned this new approach to pain about 10 years after my last surgery. I had been getting weekly bodywork treatments. My understanding of the interactions between my body and emotions was just awakening, and with it my comfort and mobility were improving. On a weekend retreat in Yosemite National Park I was invited to go on a walk with a group of friends. I was assured it would be easy and not too long. At that time I often had hip pain following my shifts as a restaurant hostess, which required lots of walking. It was also a time in my life when I had abandoned a long–held dream, thus I was not supporting my creative intellectual nature. Here again is an example of how unconsciously failing to "support" myself was coincident with increased hip pain.

The leaders of the "walk" miscalculated. Soon we were tromping through the woods with no trail – and no idea what lay ahead. We climbed through the forest for a couple of hours. To get back we had to descend a granite face (fortunately, not sheer). This whole adventure was both rewarding and harrowing for me. I could not possibly turn back, so I proceeded, reassuring myself all the way that I could do it. (One of my favorite stories as a child was The Little Engine that Could... "I think I can, I think I can, I think I can...") I got through the hike okay, all five miles of it. But, when I got into bed I could feel the faint and familiar tremors of stiffness and pain that always left me incapacitated by morning. I dreaded those feelings.

For the first time in my life I decided that I might have a choice about how my body felt. I tried an experiment in the name of personal science. First, I began to pay deep attention to my hip. I could feel the tension and fatigue gripping my bones. I knew if I allowed the tightness to remain it would constrict my circulation and reduce the healthy bathing of my muscles. I talked to my muscles, telling them they didn't have to hurt – that I could rest tomorrow. I put a gentle hand on my leg. I used the sound of the nearby river to imagine the tension being carried away. Primarily, I tried to believe in my body's health and hoped for something new to happen. To my amazement, I had no pain the next day.

Research replicates my experience. As mentioned in Chapter Four, Dr. John Kabat-Zinn at the University of Massachusetts Medical School, conducts a highly respected pain control and stress reduction program founded on the meditation principle of mindfulness. This principle demonstrates that simple, objective attention to the body, just as I discovered, can greatly reduce pain and stress. His research results are impressive. In a follow-up study conducted four years after participation in the clinic program, 67% rated their experience between 8–10 on a 1–10 scale. Of the participants, 43% said that 80–100% of their pain improvement was due to what they had learned in the program. In another study, he compared two groups of pain patients, those in his meditation program plus conventional medical care and those receiving only conventional pain treatments. The control group of non-meditators showed little change, while the meditators showed major improvements in pain, mood and psychological distress. Dr. Kabat-Zinn concluded that "These results suggest that doing something for yourself, as the people in the stress clinic were doing by engaging in meditation practice in addition to receiving medical treatment for pain can result in many positive changes that might not occur with medical treatment alone."[4]

Investigate your fear

Is your fear, the premonition of pain, warning you of a true danger or, is your fear based on memories of bad times, which may or may not be accurate?

These are important questions. I will refer to the first fear as "objectively based fear," and the second as "subjectively based fear." Subjectively based fear is wily, often fooling us into believing that there is a "clear and present danger." This inner fear can wear many masks, among them:

Comparison/judgement, the fear of not being "as good as."

Guilt, the fear of our power, our actions and inactions.

Anger, the fear of the pain of violation.

One of life's lessons is to learn to see past these veils of illusion, despite their convincing nature. Fear can make us brittle and impermeable, engaging us in unnecessary struggle. When we begin to understand the difference between fantasy and reality, we can minimize the effect of our subjective fears. We free up our energy to address the true obstacles and allow the illusory threats to blow past us in the wind.

Normal fears

During her early recovery, Judith coped with several fears both objective and subjectively based. Her surgery was very complex, requiring a significant bone graft, which was held by two wires. The wires were somewhat fragile. Judith's doctor impressed upon her the importance of the wires in her healing. She was afraid to break them, so she was extremely careful in her movements. In this case, her fear was of a real and present threat. She addressed it head on, giving care to her actions. She took responsibility. One wire did break, but due to her responsible approach the remaining wire held the graft in place long enough for it to set. She turned her initial fear into watchfulness, thus using her warning system wisely.

Judith began experiencing another fear as she approached the six- month mark after surgery. She was worried about a pulling sensation and mild discomfort in the inner thigh of her healing leg. In one of our sessions I encouraged her to give close attention to the sensations, without trying to clutch them or push them away. When she was able to feel attentive, I asked her to explore her associated thoughts and emotions. She spoke of how confident and balanced she recently felt when walking with the lift in her shoe. A sense of gloom and dread occurred without the lift to balance her. This imbalance reminded her of how she felt *six months after her previ-*

ous surgery when the artificial hip socket began to migrate out of place, creating severe problems. This was a very upsetting thought. *But just a thought.* (All of her check–ups confirmed she was healing well.)

I explained to her how her present neurological experience of imbalance could remind her body of the past experience and trigger the state-dependent associations of fear and discomfort. We talked about how the difference she felt between balance and imbalance in the present did not have to mean the same thing that it had before. She was relieved to have a new view of her feelings and reported that her leg felt much better. A few days later she realized that this time her artificial socket had been anchored with screws to insure stability, a fact she had not remembered in her state of anxiety. A visit to the doctor a few days later confirmed that she was fine. This second example shows how our subjectively based fears can pull us out of present reality and even contribute to our pain, due to the increased tensions.

Investigate your depression

How can I gather the energy to resolve my depression?

When depression descends on us, we forget that we have alternatives for solving its real or imagined challenges. We lose energy. We forget that some new bit of information could reverse our feelings of domination. We forget that our fears may have *no* basis in fact. We forget that we have untapped inner and outer resources, so we give up.

The expression – *and even the awareness* – of that powerful and often righteous emotion, anger, is often shrouded in depression. We lie to ourselves that we have no power to change. We forget to love and stand up for ourselves. Our depression may be based in our thoughts or have physiological factors that need to be addressed; in either case, we must take action to break out of the pattern.

I reached a very low point during a protracted divorce. After 18 months of negotiating I had given up all hope of resolution. I spent my time dazed and in tears, in utter despair. By chance, I met a self-defense teacher whose mission in life is to help women feel strong. I took a few much-needed lessons. Learning how to defend myself physically gave me the emotional strength to defend myself in the divorce proceedings. I replaced my passive lawyer with someone whose reputation commanded the respect of my former husband's attorney. We settled within six weeks.

I had forgotten, or I had never learned, that I could and *must* stand up for myself. This goes back to the earlier discussion of support. When we learn to support ourselves, despair can lift. Our sense of competency returns. That is why it is so important to be an active participant in your health care – and in your whole life! *Life is not a dress rehearsal, it is the premiere performance.* Depression occurs when we abandon life and ourselves, when we lie to ourselves, and when we refuse to take ourselves and our lives seriously.

Action can also be taken on the physiological factors of depression. For example, a client had been plagued with severe pre-menstrual depressions for several years. After sorting through all the possible emotional aspects, she turned to acupuncture treatments and food supplements. Her symptoms were significantly relieved in the very next cycle. That cyclic depression was clearly physiological.

A significant number of depressions need some kind of physiologically oriented care. What concerns me is that the push for a chemical panacea will end up drugging people unnecessarily. Conventional medicine still does not pay adequate attention to nutritional factors. Traditional Chinese medicine and herbology should also be considered valuable therapies. Although this book focuses on depression as a response to traumatic experiences, which set up negative thought patterns, we must remember to approach depression from every angle until we find the key, to insure that we are not leaving some aspect behind.

The key to thriving

Orphaned or abandoned infants experience deep despair and depression. The landmark research findings, referred to in Chapter Two, observed babies' failure to thrive is often due to lack of loving attention. WE *adults fail to thrive when we stop loving and attending to ourselves*. Babies have few resources to remedy their plight; they are truly dependent. But as adults, *we can act* to give ourselves what we need. It takes time to learn what we truly need, because most of us have not been taught how to care for ourselves, as discussed in earlier chapters. However, with compassionate attention to the still small voice inside, *we can learn*. Methods of learning to hear and care for yourself will be discussed at length in Chapters Six and Seven.

Another distinction is important, as Mick Jagger reminds us in his song, "You can't always get what you want, but if you try, you get what you need." What we think we *want* may be hollow in healing our depression. Many high-powered Yuppies, disillusioned with the wealth they thought would satisfy them, are turning to more modest and balanced lifestyles. With all of us, it takes time and commitment to hear our inner voice tell us what will nourish us. In the end the solution may be simple, although what is simple is not necessarily easy.

Beth's story

Beth came to me with a story that combines all the elements of this chapter. After several years of intense pain, Beth, a 35 year old mother of three children under 8 years old, learned that she needed major reconstructive hip surgery to correct an arthritic condition. The problem developed due to complications from childhood surgeries for congenital hip dislocation. Beth was frightened at the thought of surgery because of many pain- and fear-filled memories from childhood. Pain control procedures were quite different then; inadequate, bordering on cruel. She was left with extremely negative associations with anything medical. She went into counseling to prepare herself for surgery. In therapy she discovered she was also afraid that her husband would not appreciate her vulnerabilities – physical and emotional. They worked on her concerns together, as a family. He and the children made some good changes, becoming more sensitive and respectful of Beth. She learned to express her needs more clearly. By the time the surgery came Beth was feeling much more secure and supported.

The surgery went well and Beth's need for emotional support was answered. Yet, she was very hesitant to extend herself physically. She feared more pain and thus limited her activity in order to stay below the threshold that might threaten her comfort. Beth resisted her doctor's encouragement to get up and move around with her crutches. As discussed in Chapter Four, the neurological representation in the brain of an inactive limb will shrink, thus reducing coordination. One day while in the kitchen, in an unusual moment out of her wheelchair, Beth fell. She was not badly hurt, but her pain increased and she took to her bed depressed, her fears confirmed.

Beth gradually continued her recovery, now more fearful. When her doctor happily announced she was ready to use only one crutch she entered a personal crisis. Memories of childhood losses emerged, the death of her father being most vivid. She wisely returned to therapy. Her depression lifted as she came to see and understand the mosaic of forces operating. She discovered that her resistance to recovering physically was directly related to the fear that if she became strong and capable her husband would no longer respect and care for her feelings of vulnerability. This was a legitimate concern. Her husband had grown up with deep seated patterns of denial and lack of awareness in his family. Personal vulnerabilities – physical or emotional – simply did not exist in his thinking. Initially, he was more attentive to her after surgery. However, as time went on he became more distant again, awakening her fears of abandonment, related to the death of her father.

This case demonstrates how essential it is to be aware and respectful of one's experience. A very important marital dynamic that could break the marriage was revealed. They addressed it partially before the surgery, but clearly something inside Beth needed the subject brought up again. It is a tremendous gift to have this type of situation show so clearly a more basic problem. Beth's adversity, as well as her pain, fear and depression, was an opportunity to grow. She took the time and care necessary to identify and address the deeper issues:

- Her pain was not as bad as she feared, and she did use it as a tool to go deeper into her life experience.

- Her fear of her husband's lack of awareness was legitimate.

- Her depression lifted when she took action.

Both Beth's body and her marriage will be stronger because of her courage to look inside, face her fears and to call upon her husband to face his own fears about vulnerability.

Working through a fall

No one around Beth at the time of her fall knew how to help her. She had to piece it together for herself over many months. (I was not working with her at the time.) When a client I am working with takes a fall I deal with it in several ways. We talk about exactly how the fall happened, the place, how they were using their body and any other specifics, so that the client understands and can learn to avoid future falls. Together we give gentle physical attention to the uncomfortable area, being attentive to emotional associations. This often relieves the immediate discomfort. Attentiveness can also allow the kinds of fears or other insights, similar to Beth's, to emerge. Finally, the client and I examine and refine how they are walking and moving. By the time the client leaves my office she understands what happened physically and emotionally, feels more comfortable physically and can now give her attention to new details in how she moves. Fear and depression dissolve when we become aware and use information within and around us.

Dissolving the triangle

When we can see the pattern clearly, our personal Bermuda Triangle loses its mystery (Figure 5.1). To dissolve the triangle, find a quiet inner place, not judging, not hysterical. Be patient. A quiet mind allows the storm clouds to settle. Consider this inverted triangle, it is precarious. Imagine how you could begin to dismantle this structure by choosing one corner and addressing it directly. Choose one part, instead of trying to take on all three aspects of the triangle at once. The pattern will be broken when one corner is removed. This simple model can be very useful in catching yourself and bringing yourself back into balance.

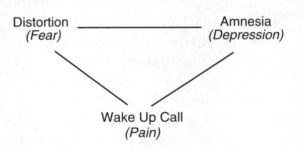

Distortion   Amnesia
(Fear)   (Depression)

Wake Up Call
(Pain)

Figure 5.1 The Bermuda Triangle

Pain is a wake-up call to activate our tools of self-protection and repair.

Pain triggers our basic fears of mortality. In one instance, I thought (was afraid) I would quite literally die of the pain when my husband left me. Fortunately, I have since learned that my emotional pain is often based on misunderstanding reality, or confusing the present with past pain. I can cause my own emotional pain by not seeing my situation clearly and practically. Similarly, physical pain is worsened by fear and its bodily manifestations of constriction and alarm. It is not hard to slip into thinking "this pain is killing me." That belief is a misunderstanding which will undermine our ability to cope constructively. Pain, in any form, can be horrible and seem unbearable, but it is only sensation. Pain is not lethal. It is a call to look at our situation and find the tools to change things. Quite often the tools are inside us, just waiting to be discovered and developed.

Fear is distortion, thoughts of the past projected onto the present and future.

In my personal and professional work I have seen that the fear of something is always worse than the actual dreaded sensation or task. Fear is an illusion based on past experiences that may or may not even be accurately remembered. Fear can cripple us, by causing the loss of trust and abandonment of hope. We may expect to be weak, imbalanced and to endure pain "forever." We worry that "the worst" will keep happening; that our hip will "fall apart," that more surgery will be necessary, that our life will always be consumed by the negative experiences. The restrictions generated by fear can wither our relationships with our body, our emotions, other people and our outer world. It is our responsibility to stay in the present and know what is real, moment to moment if necessary, to correct the distortions.

Depression is amnesia, forgetting the resources of our true selves.

One of my most useful and accessible tools is remembering that depression is self-abandonment. But why do we abandon ourselves? For me, the self-abandonment is due to fear that I cannot correct, get out of, transcend or overcome the crisis I feel. When I take a moment to look around and recognize my options, it is fear of my own helplessness – an unfounded fear – that brings on depression. Remembering that we have choices and the possibility to take action removes that sense of helplessness and breaks the grip of depression.

Questions like these will help identify the concerns below the surface of your awareness:

Pain:

• How can I comfort or relax myself?

• What do I need to listen to inside?

• What can I learn from this pain?

Fear:

• Is my anger a mask of fear?

• Is my self-punishment the voice of fear, trying to stop me from making further "mistakes?"

• Is my fear making me rigid, emotionally and/or physically, and closed off to possible solutions?

Depression:

• How am I abandoning myself?

• What am I forgetting?

• What action can I take for myself?

When you give care to one corner of the triangle, the structure creating the downward spiral will weaken and you will discover your ability to move forward. Any time we are faced with the unknown it is natural to be a bit wary. It is smart to be vigilant. We must also be aware of the treacherous triangle of pain, fear and depression and how it seeks to perpetuate itself through bait-and-switch games and feelings of confusion and despair. Step by step, you learn how and what you need to do to diffuse this cycle. Just like training a puppy, consistency and patience are essential.

Conclusion

Healing begins when you let go of what is not true in the present. This allows you to trust your perceptions, realize you have choices and learn new ways to live in your body. Your doubts and fears made you forget that your life, your opportunity and your power is in the present moment. Rachael Naomi Remen, M.D., pioneer in humanizing the medical profession, states that "Health becomes the freedom not to react to things, but to respond and have many different options – not to be trapped by an old belief about life." In the following chapters I will discuss specific ways to develop and maintain a new approach to yourself and your health. I encourage you to read the whole book first, then go back to the practices that most interest you.

Chapter 6

Listening to the River

The more you know yourself, the more clarity there
is. Self knowledge has no end – you don't come to an
achievement, you don't come to a conclusion.
It is an endless river.

– Krishnamurti

THIS CHAPTER PROVIDES A VARIETY OF TOOLS for increasing your emotional awareness and self-knowledge. Finding your balance after surgery or injury includes observing and accepting how the physical trauma affected you emotionally. Knowing what you feel below the surface clears your mind of unnecessary static and guards against emotions stifling your flexibility and health. We each have our own rhythms and preferences. There is no right or wrong way to proceed. I have included several techniques so that you can discover what suits your taste...or you can invent your own. The key to emotional awareness is taking the time to listen to your inner process with respect and appreciation – a little humor doesn't hurt, either.

Return to your body

The foundation of my training for hands-on work with people is the Rosen Method of bodywork, which is based on the principle that relaxation is the gateway to awareness.[1] I learned to use my hands in a gentle and receptive way, to encourage a sense of safety.

Creating a background of safety allows relaxation and recollection of memories held in the body. These memories may come in the form of images, thoughts, emotions or simple physical releases as I described my own experience in Chapter Two. Our bodies seem to be the last hold-outs in the personal growth process. We can intellectually understand our situations, but until we have *felt* the feelings in our bodies, experienced the *physical insight,* we may remain stuck.

Conversely, chronic tensions in the body may point to unresolved emotions. Very early in my career, while working as a masseuse in a women's health club, a woman came to see me with severe stiffness in her neck and shoulders. The stiffness started after a traffic accident. In a flat, detached tone she told me how a motorcyclist had hit her car head-on and been killed. As she spoke, she held her arms out stiff as if bracing herself against the steering wheel of a car. She said she really didn't have any feelings about the experience.

However, her body was frozen in a braced position. It was as if the accident had lodged in her body, not allowing her to forget, try as she might, to ignore the depth of the experience in which another person died in front of her.

The recognition of my body's role in expressing my life experience drew me away from my conventional psychological training to study bodymind dynamics. The stories my clients told me strengthened my conviction that the interplay of the body and mind had to be respected and addressed. The following is my favorite description of how I use my hands when working with a client; my goal is to create another way of communicating.

I was giving Keith a sample of my work as we sat in front of the TV. He was the husband of a friend and it was the first time I had met him. He had done two tours of duty in Viet Nam, which had left him with a rough exterior. Within a few minutes of touching his flannel-shirted shoulders as he drank a beer, he said quietly, *"You're listening with your hands."* Yes, I realized, that was what I was doing. It had never been articulated so simply or so beautifully. I learned that Keith had studied Buddhist meditation while in Viet Nam, which he said kept him together, body and soul, and made him highly sensitive.

You can learn to listen to your own body with your hands. It is a way of returning to the beginning, when your nonverbal experience was primary. As a baby, your first experience of the world is tactile. You explored your world with your hands, expressed yourself with your whole body. Your body continues to register all your experiences, whether you express them physically or not. Listening with your hands is a gentle way of giving your body a voice.

Listening with your hands

Place your hands gently on the part of your body that calls for attention – perhaps your injured/operated part, or your heart. Let the skin of your hands reach out for the skin of that part of your body. Allow a safe connection with this part of yourself that is in need of attention. You don't have to *do* anything, just touch yourself with a present, friendly hand. Be attentive, as if you are listening to a very soft spoken person who is just learning to express him or herself in a new language. Be patient, have an open mind and an open heart.

This may open the door for feelings or insights. Allow whatever is there to emerge, without judgment. Your experience may be complete in itself, or it may bring up thoughts you would like to follow-up yourself or with a therapist. This is a tool I continue to use for comfort and insight. The next section will provide tools for further exploration.

Subpersonalities

Almost everyone I know has a familiar group of conflicting voices that resound in their head. Expressions such as, "On one hand I feel this way, but on the other hand...," "I'm in two minds about that" and "I don't know what got into me" all acknowledge this multiplicity within. Some of these voices are very distinct, even predictable. Other inside pressures are vague. Sometimes it can seem that we are possessed by a parent, an ornery teenager, a frightened child, or a harsh critic, just to name a few. There is also great wisdom to be found within when we listen.

Psychology is full of theories that describe this common experience. Freud was a pioneer with his theory of the id, ego

and superego. Jung described inner complexes and arche-
types. Transactional Analysis presents Adult, Parent and
Child parts of self. Gestalt therapy "invites you to invade
your own privacy" and discover the parts of yourself that you
rejected for "causing too much trouble" during a time of
stress. Research examining Multiple Personality Disorder
suggest that we are all "multiples", but that pathology arises
when the boundaries become disturbed.[2]

A good example of this natural tendency happened to me
as I wrote the paragraph above. A voice grumbled "This is
stupid, you don't know how to say what you mean...they'll
never understand this...or accept it...you can't write...give it
up...*ad nauseam.*" Sound familiar? This is how our fear of
criticism attempts to influence us and inhibit us. Usually self
"protection" is the root – a voice of the past trying to "save"
us from replaying some past humiliation or danger. As discussed in Chapter Five, fear is based on past, not present.
I find it very useful to "flesh out" these voices so that I can
better understand what is going on inside of me and move
forward with a clear sense of purpose. Here's how I do it:

Listening to your inner dialog

Take some time to listen to yourself (or selves!). Stop reading.
What messages come to mind? Observe... Choose one and
give it you full attention. What wants to be heard? What is
the tone of voice?...See the source of the voice in your imag-
ination...What does it look like?... How is it dressed?... Is it
familiar to you, like you were at a younger age, or does it
seem like a different person? Allow the full character to
emerge, just as if you were a playwright creating a character.

Writing a dialog between your conscious self and the inner
voice can be a powerful way to unlock doors bursting with in-

sight. It may feel a little artificial at first, but be patient and open to getting the flow moving. The process often takes on a feeling of meditation or automatic writing. Just trust it and see where it leads, you may be surprised. The following describes one of my experiences.

In my personal work I have given a lot of attention to the "children" inside me who went through medical treatment and surgery. For example, I know that some of my former feelings of restriction stem directly from spending most of my first 18 months of life in a full-body cast. While writing this book I reached a period of confusion. I used this process of inner dialog during a gestalt therapy session to break through the fog and unexpectedly discovered my true motivation for writing. It is a good example of how one loose thread of thought can lead to a tapestry of subconscious associations. The same technique can be done alone, writing or speaking aloud:

When I became quiet and went inside I was aware of the emotional pain about a men's group my former husband had started with our "mutual" male friends when he left our marriage. First I was filled with voiceless, helpless feelings. Then I asked myself, Who is the voiceless one? *"Three in casts"* was the answer. I waited and the three ages I was in body casts came into my mind. I talked to them one by one.

First, I thought about myself as an infant in the cast. I imagined the feeling of restriction in the concrete-like plaster. I remembered pictures of myself at that time, and the stories that I had heard. I took myself "there" in every way I could. I observed myself at that time, as if I were watching a movie. I waited...I felt no need from my baby self to communicate to me as an adult...I waited again, then I was compelled to tell that baby, *"I am writing my book for you."* With that, I felt complete with that time in my life.

Next I thought of myself at ten years old. I put myself there. I became very ill after surgery at that age. I developed an infection in the operated hip, lost weight and had to be re-hospitalized. I was so sensitive that any movement, like a bump to my bed, caused pain. I was stoic at the time, known as a "good patient." Inside I was in deep despair. From my present perspective I felt great compassion for this child. I recalled my suicidal feelings at 10 and 11 years old. I saw no hope and the doctors gave me no reassurance. I was compelled to say to that 10 year old, *"I'm glad you didn't give up."*...I found myself rubbing "her back" (a pillow that happened to be in front of me). I repeated over and over,"...*it turned out okay...I'm okay now...Look how strong and beautiful I am."* When I felt a sense of peace I moved on.

When I returned to my self at the age of 12 I found an angry and callous character. She *"knew that the Doctors didn't know what they were doing,"* but she wasn't about to give up, even though she was stuck in plaster from armpit to toes. She said forcefully, *"I won't go away...I am not helpless, I will make them listen!"* From the present I felt compelled to talk to her about how the surgeon had removed a muscle he decided was of no use. I told the angry 12 year old, *"I am sorry about what they did to you: the 'soft tissue release'* (surgical term for cutting tangled scar and muscle tissue with a knife). *That's what I now do with my hands, with touch. Tight muscles or damaged muscles don't have to be cut. That will never happen to us again. I promise."* I was catapulted from there to the doctors who had treated me, and said to them,

"You need to understand that immobilization of the body damages the person's self-perception and their perception of reality...The most current brain/body research shows that is true...I know it from experience...when a limb is immobilized the corresponding place in the brain is usurped by other, more active parts of the body...Please learn this neurology, learn new ways to treat people. Self-concept is critical to recovery and immobilization obscures that."

In reference to the removal of one my hip flexing muscles:... *"There is no junk in the body. You cannot cut creatively and not cause ripple effects. We are each given only one body, one full set of parts, we need them all – think of this before you cut."* This was an impassioned plea for greater awareness on the part of the medical profession, greater thought given to how the treatment of the body affects the psyche – which will in turn affect the body. All of this was very emotional, so I took time to rest.

As I rested, I realized that the thoughtlessness of my "friends" participating in the men's group triggered my early feelings of voicelessness and victimization at the hands of a more powerful group of thoughtless men, the small group of doctors who had in fact been dangerous to me. It was completely rational to feel threatened and at the doctors' mercy – three in particular placed me in real peril.

I closed my eyes and went inside again...With each child listened to and cared for, I saw them, one by one, slip out of their casts...in my last image, spontaneously we four joined hands in a circle to dance.

Your most important tools for working with yourself in this way are an open mind, curiosity, compassion, patience and courage. You will not remember anything that is "too much" for you to handle. Approach this exercise with kindness and the knowledge that you are here, safe in the present now. The steps are simple and can be written, visualized or spoken:

1. *Listen to yourself.* I begin with closing my eyes, sitting comfortably and paying attention to my body. As I quiet myself, I notice what sensations or thoughts call my attention. If I have a persistent physical feeling I stay with it...allow it to expand and imagine what it would say if it had a voice.

2. *Accept whatever comes up.* I accept whatever comes up as a clue. I may not understand it yet, but I am willing to play with it, follow it for a bit – until it runs out of juice. Often the real issues are overlaid by immediate and sometimes nonsensical thoughts or associations. Patience and open-minuteness pay off.

3. *Be curious and creative.* I ask lots of questions; Who/what inside me has this feeling?...What made them feel that?...What is the story that needs to come into the light?

4. *Allow the story to unfold.* Allow the story to reel out, like fishing line. The unconscious has its own currents that often do not follow linear patterns. Patience and a bit of self-indulgence facilitate the flow.

5. *Notice how this story plays out in other situations in your life.* Does this story sound familiar? Are there simi-

larities to other times in your life? What can you learn to ease and improve your ways of handling these situations?

The example I used was working with my "inner children." The same process can be applied to working with the voices of fear, judgment and whatever else you encounter. My clients and I find it very beneficial to give the injured part of the body a voice, just like a character. Follow the trail back to the deepest roots of the emotions, like a detective. Not interpreting from some theory, but discovering what is there from a compassionate and common sense perspective.

Related techniques

Writing. Stream of consciousness writing helps to unblock a variety of problems: anger, pain, confusion or whatever. Let the words flow with no concern for grammar or spelling. Just get those thoughts and feelings out of your head and onto the paper where you can see them objectively.

Artwork. Drawing, sculpting or collage unveils inner understanding, nonverbally. You can start with a topic in mind, or not. It's fun and interesting to let your hands speak to you through form and image. Expressing how your body feels or would like to feel is a good use of these media.

Each of these methods encourage appreciation and respect of *all* aspects of your self. Each aspect evolved for a reason which was adaptive *at the time* and needs acknowledgment before it will become dormant. Re-acquainting yourself with these parts, perhaps making friends and correcting misunderstandings, gives honor to all that is you. Simply trying to reject or amputate a unpopular quality requires an attack on yourself, which generally is neither instructive or effective.

Acknowledging your pain or fear begins the process of insight and release.

Meditation

Meditation is the art of taming your thoughts, observing without getting involved. It has been practiced in many forms throughout history and across cultures. The benefits of a quiet mind, which fosters a quiet body, are universal. Meditation is simple, but not necessarily easy. The mind is a busy place, as described in the section above. Mediation is another way to deal with our mental hubbub.

Basic meditation

Begin by giving yourself at least 10 minutes of sitting. As you incorporate meditation into your life, you will find that you naturally meditate longer, and the time passes more quickly.

Choose a quiet place that will be your meditation spot. You may want to mark it somehow, with flowers, a candle, or anything that has special meaning to you. Creating a sense of the sacred – whatever that means to you – is a way of honoring this process of self-care.

Choose a time when you can be alone, with the house quiet. Unplug the phone. Some people get up before the rest of the household rises to insure privacy. Make sure you will have no distractions during your time with yourself.

Sit comfortably, with your back in a dignified and self-supporting position, in a straight backed chair or on a floor cushion. I find it useful to start my meditation with a short invocation that I have used every time I meditate for many years. You may wish to say a short prayer or affirmation. It could be as simple as "I set this time aside for my own well-being." Try something on for size, as a way of settling yourself and setting a tone. Observing the in flow and out flow of your breath is a useful anchor for focusing your attention in the present. Then sit back and watch the show. You may feel aches, become restless, think of things obscure or "urgent." All of these are characteristics of what the Buddhists call "the monkey mind." Continue to just watch and breathe, for these 10 minutes there is nothing to do.

This is not a time to think about things. It is a time to *not* think. Just observe your thoughts, like leaves floating past you on a river. It is a time to allow thoughts and feelings to emerge and *not* follow them, *not* try to figure them out, *not* indulge them or try to solve them. It is a time to just watch...and as you do this, over time, you will find you are watching from a different place. You are developing your observing self that can be detached from all the "stuff" of the mind. It is the part of you that can see and accept What Is – not What Might Be, What Should Be, What Has Been – simply what is true for you in this moment. You will discover the benefits of this.[3]

Imagery

Imagery can be defined as how thought awakens and uses the senses; hearing, sight, touch, smell, taste and movement. Take a moment to recall how you feel when you hear your favorite song, smell your favorite food, or imagine the touch of your lover. You are experiencing the communication between perception, emotion and physiology. According to Dr. Jeanne Achterberg, one of the leaders in clinical research in the uses of imagery, "The image is the world's oldest and greatest healing resource." It is a tool in modern medicine and indigenous healing practices alike. The benefits of imagery have been validated in the treatment of chronic pain, cancer, diabetes, bone growth, burn injury, rheumatoid arthritis, as well as stress-related symptoms such as migraine headaches and hypertension, and during childbirth.

The general research findings conclude:

1. Images relate to physiological states;

2. Images may either precede or follow physiological changes, indicating both a causative and reactive role;

3. Images can be induced by conscious, deliberate behavior, as well as by subconscious acts (electrical stimulation of the brain, reverie, dreaming, etc.);

4. Images can be considered as the hypothetical bridge between conscious processing of information and physiological change;

5. Images can exhibit influence over the voluntary nervous system, as well as the involuntary nervous system (internal organs and systems thought to be beyond our conscious influence).[4]

These research findings underline the mind-body interaction from another perspective. They document that imagery is a powerful tool. Olympic athletes and other peak performers use imagery extensively to rehearse and enhance every detail of their chosen task. You can too, in any aspect of your life.

The possibilities are endless. You already use imagery everyday without thinking about it. For example, when you control your bladder with the unconscious image of a nearby comfort station. You might as well use it consciously for your health and well-being. It is important for any use of imagery to make it as real as you can, activating all your senses to create the experience within. When using imagery in your health care, study the basic anatomy and elements of your treatment procedures. You don't need to know exactly how the healing occurs, but understanding the basics is beneficial. It's like ordering food in a restaurant: know what you want, but you don't have to go into the kitchen and instruct the chef how to prepare the meal.

Here's a sample imagery exercise.

For body part replacement

To begin, settle yourself in a comfortable resting position – reclining or sitting. Be sure you are truly comfortable, take time arranging yourself to be just right. Close your eyes.

Imagine the part of your body that is diseased and is scheduled to be replaced (If the replacement has already been completed imagine your original anatomy) ...Allow any thoughts or feelings to come to mind, even if they seem silly. Talk to that part about whatever comes up....Let your body talk to you...listen to it...Remember to thank it for its service to you, despite the problems. Explain why it is now necessary for a new part to take on its role. Some people find that seeing the retired or resting part in a safe environment, rewarded for its efforts, is comforting and makes it easier to say good-bye.

Next, imagine the area of your body with the new part. See the new part there, perfectly in place. Imagine your blood bathing it...your tissues knitting it into themselves...allow the boundaries to dissolve between you and the "new"...know that your body's intelligence will teach this new addition all it needs to know to participate fully in the everyday functioning of your body...Love it for its role in maintaining and improving your quality of life...Love it, for it is now you. See and feel yourself as whole, moving easily and comfortably.

Yield to the imagery. Whenever your feelings are in conflict with your image, the dominant feelings will prevail. If you have doubts or resistance, look at them — they are probably the shadows of fear. Take the risk to set your fears aside and be open to something different. Give yourself the chance for a new beginning.

Your autobiography

One of the best tools I have found for self-awareness is writing an autobiography. Up till now, I have emphasized non-intellectual ways to experience yourself. The autobiography is the most "thinking" tool I suggest. I encourage you to use your tools of physical and emotional awareness to enrich your storytelling. With increased sensory awareness and personal clarity, gained by examining your life, your options and your power to make changes in your life increase. Possibilities for self-care and life choices expand when your self-understanding deepens. Taking the time to sit down and reflect on your life will allow you to see patterns that link the different aspects of your experience. I have observed in myself and others that our bodies often express what we do not bring to consciousness. The process of reviewing your life will help point out which parts of your life you remember well, and which parts are dim. You may be surprised at what you learn about yourself.

Taking time out to write may seem boring or irrelevant when you are focused on improving your physical symptoms and becoming more comfortable and active. If you feel hesitant about this kind of introspection, you are quite normal. Stay with it, your resistance or apathy will help slow down the pace of your life in preparation for the necessary reflection. The reward is worth it. You will be moving in a new direction and into a new relationship to yourself during the quiet moments when it looks like you are doing nothing. This is a very valuable time, indeed. Great richness will follow.

As Nancy Anderson suggests in her book, Work With Passion, start by describing the family you were born into. Include your grandparents. Describe each member's beliefs about health, gender roles, spirituality and/or religion, children, work, and money. Take your time reviewing your early childhood, school years, young adulthood up to the present. Include all injuries, illnesses or surgeries. Review the emotional challenges you faced, such as moving, loss of a loved one (including pets), school experiences. Anderson suggests that you refer to your family members by their first names, rather than their titles of "Mom", "Dad" and so on. She urges that you honor your own timing as you write and include the sensations, emotions and insights that come to you as you go along. Her book offers the most complete approach to autobiography I have found. She uses it in her work as a career consultant as the first step to helping her clients find the work that they love, how they can support themselves in a way they care about and enjoy.

Compassionate action

The ability to comfort yourself is an important partner for self-awareness. It is essential that you are able to show loving respect for your own needs. This skill allows you to be happier when you are alone and a clearer, independent partner in your relationships. Self-care is acting on what you have learned by listening to your inner voice. With yourself, it may take the form of resting or withdrawing when you need to, taking a hot bath, giving yourself a special treat or reaching out for help. With others, self-care can take the form of saying what you really need to say, regardless of how clumsy or awkward you feel, and having compassion for yourself through the process. Since most of us did not learn to truly take care of ourselves, your attempts in learning may feel strange, even embarrassing. You will become better with practice. The following is one way to show compassion for your self.

Cradling

This practice provides a structure for simple self-encouragement and comfort. It has roots in both the Basque and African cultures. The woman I learned it from called it "cradling." This is useful to do before going to sleep, or at any time when you are feeling ragged. Gently hugging yourself, or placing your hands on your heart as you review the day adds to the benefits.

Simply take time to reflect on your day and on yourself by answering these questions, putting all judgments aside:

1. Which of my strengths do I chose to honor today?

2. What do I like about myself in this moment?

3. What have I, or am I, contributing to my world?

4. What love have I given or received today?

Answering these questions will help you find the light in the darkness you may have focused on during the day. It is a way of regaining your perspective and nurturing your strengths.

Conclusion

All of the techniques I have discussed in this chapter encourage mindfulness, defined by Harvard Professor Ellen Langer as;

1. the creation of new categories,

2. openness to new information, and

3. awareness of more than one perspective.[5]

Acting from the perspective of your habitual set of thoughts and behaviors limits you to "solutions" of the past. Mindfulness gives you the opportunity to live your life awake and creatively engaged with all that is within you and around you, opening new doors to well being. The next chapter takes mindfulness into movement, enriching your tool kit of self-care.

Self in Motion

And in that moment, when the body became action,
the leg, the flesh became quick and alive,
the flesh became music, incarnate solid music.
All of me, body and soul, became music in that moment.

– Oliver Sacks
<u>A Leg to Stand On</u>

L IFE IS MOVEMENT. WITHIN US AND AROUND US
there is constant movement of molecules – air,
fluids, solids – each touching and being touched. Each
encounter is new. Just as the flow of traffic can become congested, we may stop the movement within
ourselves. This is especially true when our body has
been injured or violated. There is a natural tendency
to protect the traumatized area, to hold it still. This
may be useful immediately following the trauma, but
often the body "forgets" to release when the danger

has passed. Chronic tensions and fear create blocks to movement and circulation. Careful attention helps us to discover
our inner points of gridlock, opening avenues to the natural
flow of movement.

Trauma or lack of use causes the body to forget its natural
ease in movement. Often movement patterns form to avoid
pain or compensate for weakness. Fear is a very active element of these patterns. Remember that fear is a reaction to
past experiences; trust is openness to the freshness of the
present. Following surgery, it is natural to return to familiar,
often fearful patterns – even though they are no longer relevant. It is never too late to establish fresh, more balanced
ways of moving. (I did not begin my exploration of compli-
mentary approaches to improving my comfort and mobility
until 10 years after my last surgery.) The purpose of the
movement practices I describe in this chapter is to introduce
safe and novel situations in which you can discover new possibilities. The intelligence of your nervous system will re-as-
sert itself through movement and alignment in more efficient,
comfortable and supportive patterns. I learned this approach
to movement through my study of Eutony.[1] Simplicity and
awareness are the keys.

Basic knowledge of anatomy enhances the movement practices, just like a road map helps to orient you to a new locale.
I will include some anatomical information with the movement descriptions. Popular culture emphasizes muscles, ne-
glecting our equally important skin and skeletal systems.
Your skin is critical to circulation and nervous system organization, for example. An accurate body image includes
knowledge of the nature and shapes of your bones. Throughout your body, your bones are shaped to help you move (as
introduced in Chapter Three). Study an anatomy book – you

may be amazed. Awareness of the natural forms that actually initiate movement will lighten and increase your mobility. For example, the back of your thigh bone is gently arched, which facilitates the easy forward swing of your leg in walking. Appreciation of your body's organization make self-care and movement easier and more meaningful.(The Anatomy Coloring Book, by Kapit & Elson, is an excellent and inexpensive basic reference.)

It is my purpose to help you find wonder and inspiration in the physical creation you know as your body. Past experiences with surgery and the "blood and guts" emphasis in the media can create a repulsion reflex when you think about the inner workings of your body. Suspend your old images and see the systems of your body as whole, uncut by scalpels, protected from cameras, known only to you with your inner eyes.

Meeting your bones

Taking time to get to know your bones can be fun and interesting. I have also found it very beneficial. There are many contours, arches, funny knobs and mysterious crevices you can discover when you take the time. All these are intimately involved in your ease of movement and balance.

Your foot is a good place to start. (If it is difficult to reach your foot, follow the same steps exploring your hand starting with your thumb.) Begin by tracing the bones of you big toe. Gently and firmly feel for the beginning and end of each bone. You want to be able to find as much of each bone as you can. Use a curious, caring touch; don't poke or pinch yourself in uncomfortable ways. As you become more familiar, and as your muscle tone balances, your bones will be easier to locate. Sometimes tight muscles bunch up and obscure the bone from your touch. A gentle touch helps ease the tightness.

Continue exploring each of your toes, following them one by one up into the body of your foot. Trace around all sides of each bone you find. Feel how the end of one bone and the beginning of another make a space: a joint. Jiggle the joints carefully to wake up your sensitivity and flexibility. You can tap a bone gently with your finger tip or a bamboo chopstick to create a vibration. Observe the affects of the vibration. When you are finished with one foot notice if your feet feel the same or different.

You can explore your whole skeleton in this simple way. If you have an uncomfortable area of your body, explore the more comfortable side first, then gently trace the painful area. For example, if your left knee hurts, explore the right knee first. Your central nervous system will carry the experience over from right to left, preparing the left side for your touch. Tracing your bones clarifies your inner architecture, eases constrictions and wakes up the circulation of sleepy areas in your body.

Movement

I will be presenting a few simple movement practices you can use to balance and sensitize your body. These are simple practices to get you started...to *play* with...to begin the new relationship with your self, body and mind together. I have chosen specific practices that will serve to integrate your body by awakening the dynamics between your upper and lower body that may have become muted by your habitual ways of getting through life.

Approach each movement with a beginner's mind, especially when you are coming back from injury or surgery. Do not do these practices by rote. You have the opportunity *in every moment* to learn more comfortable and efficient ways of moving. You can be a detective researching your own potentials and sensitivities. You will discover what is best for you as you increase your sensitivity and understanding of your whole self. Incorporating this approach into your daily life will help you discover how you can control your own comfort.

Move through all of these practices with an attitude of openness and gentleness with yourself. This approach is very different from exercises or calisthenics. It gives you the opportunity to discover your natural movement rhythms. It is body meditation...discovering subtle information about yourself. If thoughts or emotions arise, just observe them, allow them to be present. Take time to learn about how your body and mind interact. Read each practice all the way through before you try it. Follow the cautions I mention and have your doctor check them for your specific conditions. These practices are also available on tape (see Resource section).

Lying down practices

Your skin

The skin develops from the same cell layer that forms the brain and nervous tissues in the embryo. When you touch the skin, you are touching the deepest sensory and information-processing structures of the brain. The skin and brain are like the surface and depth of a lake. Both are of the same medium and to touch the surface is to stir the depths.

In approximately one square inch of your skin there are close to 3,000,000 cells, 100 sweat glands, 50 nerve endings, 3 feet of blood vessels and nearly as much length of lymph vessels. The skin receives about one-third of the heart's output of oxygenated blood. The whole skin has approximately 640,000 sensory receptors that connect to the spinal cord through over 500,000 nerve fibers. Appreciate the richness of your inner activity as you do the following practice:

1. *Painting your skin*

This practice is excellent for a whole-body relaxation and awakening. You may be surprised at the results of this simple process.

Leave yourself a lot of time to do this practice. I have been known to spend an hour and a half, but even just a few minutes are beneficial. Wear non-binding clothes which allow you to move freely. Put the concerns of the day on hold. Unplug the phone. Be sure you are warm enough to be relaxed. Take time to settle onto the floor.

Lie on your back on a carpeted floor. Notice how your body is touching the floor. Take time to feel the surface of your skin in this resting position – the areas that are touching the rough carpet, the parts that are touching your clothes, and the parts where the air is touching your skin. Notice these different sensations. Be aware of your breathing. Take an inventory of how your body feels now, so you can compare it with how you feel after this practice.

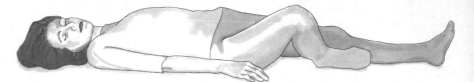

Figure 7.1 Painting Your Skin.

You will be active with one side of your body first. Choose the side that is most comfortable today. If you are recovering from trauma or surgery begin with the non-injured side. The nervous system will transfer what you do on this side to your healing side, which prepares it for later activity.

Begin to explore the floor with the heel of your foot on the side you chose. Rub your heel gently along the floor; as you do this let your body be at rest. Explore the skin of your whole foot, bending your knee or moving your leg however your need to, but with as little effort as possible, as if you were going to paint your foot with the floor. You will find yourself needing to roll to touch all the surfaces of your foot. Let your body roll easily and smoothly, feeling the support from the floor for as much of your body as possible. You can also use your other foot or knee to reach the tricky places, if you like. Every few minutes take a time to rest, let all of your activity go and allow your body to adjust to this new stimulation.

Continue gradually all the way up the side of your body – rolling and resting. Remember to let your whole body, including your head, to be supported by the floor. This is meant to be a pleasurable process, *without strain of any kind*. Allow your arms to find their natural positions as you move. Find the contours, the roundness of your body. I find that my sides and armpits always like this "floor massage." Don't be too ambitious, reach the places you can reach today, knowing that every day is different.

As you explore, remember how rich your skin is with nerves and blood vessels – *there is lots of activity going on inside you*. The inner layers of the skin's connective tissue weave through the muscles and down to the bones, forming a skin of the bone and *inside* the hollow parts of the bones.

This connective tissue forms the tendons, which attach muscle to bone and ligaments which attach bone to bone. All of this tissue is inseparable from the skin you are touching against the floor.

Move, then rest frequently to allow your nervous system to integrate. Check for your gestures of concentration: tight jaw, furrowed brow, clenched fist...get to know what habits you have that drain your energy unconsciously.

When you feel that side complete, come back to the starting position on your back and observe how you feel, compare the two sides of your body.

When you are ready, begin exploring your other foot, and gradually, the whole other side of your body, with your beginner's mind. When you finish, roll onto your back, legs extended, and reflect on what you learned about yourself. Notice how you feel now compared to how you felt when you first lay down.

Your hips

Your hips belong to the family of synovial joints, which are characterized by encapsulated space between the bones and by freedom of movement. The bones creating the joint are surrounded by a capsule made of dense fibrous connective tissue that is contiguous with the skin of the bones (periosteum). The capsule protects and strengthens the joint. Inside the capsule, the synovial membrane produces the fluid that lubricates the joint, ensuring smooth action. Other examples of synovial joints are the shoulders, fingers and joints of the spine. Movement in the joint stimulates production of the lubricating fluid; therefore, using your joints is essential to their health and flexibility. Size of the movement is less important than consistency. Even if your joints are uncomfortable, look for ways to introduce a little spring into them, keeping in mind the space between the bones. Let that image give you room to move.

2. Hip Stirring

This movement is excellent for keeping your hip joints and shoulders moving. Mobility of your hips can also help keep your back and knees comfortable. Remember that your hip is a ball-and-socket joint; think of the round, smooth surfaces you can have inside.

Lie on your back, feet flat on the floor with your knees up, arms comfortably at your sides. Position your feet so that your legs feel supported without effort. Having your feet and knees parallel is best.

Choosing the most comfortable side, easily bring your knee toward your chest and hold that knee with the same-side hand, just below the kneecap if possible. Allow your arm to be straight, so your knee is resting at arm's length...you're not gripping your knee to your chest. With your arm straight your hand supports your knee and your knee suspends your arm.

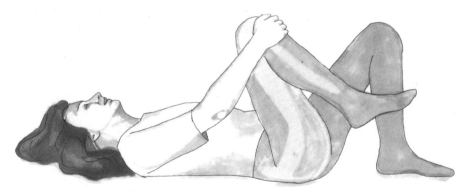

Figure 7.2 Hip Stirring.

Imagine your have a pen light on your knee. Begin to make slow, tiny circles with your knee, as if you were drawing little circles on the ceiling with the light. Keep the circles small and round, to ensure that you are rotating the round head of your femur in your hip socket. Notice where the movement occurs: it should be very deep and low in your pelvis, where your hip joint is located. A friend likened this movement to stirring the sugar at the bottom of a cup of coffee. Remember to go slow and pay attention to your movement. Do this a few times (5-10 times is fine), then reverse the direction of the circles. Be sure to keep your movements comfortable and easy at all times. Remember the space in the joints, let your shoulder and hip enjoy the roundness of the movement. Small is beautiful in this case, *the roundness, comfort and ease are the important things*. When you let your foot down gently to rest, notice how that foot is standing and observe how you feel all over.

When you are ready, do the other side.

Your hands, arms, shoulders, neck, chest and face

Each part of our body affects each other part in movement, as well as more subtle processes. The next practice mobilizes the whole upper body. You will be moving many joints, creating lots of room to move and breathe. As you begin to explore, know that there are 27 bones in each hand, two bones in your lower arms, and spaces in between all those bones. Know that there are joints where each rib meets your sternum in the front *and* your spine in the back. The image of a fixed rib "cage" is inaccurate. It's better to imagine your upper body as resembling the gills of a fish, expanding and contracting with each breath. Those who have been through heart surgery have had their whole upper torso wrenched apart. It is common for a pattern of rigidity to develop around the chest following that experience. A heart broken by emotions can cause the same body pattern. The following practice is helpful in relieving any tensions of the upper body and easing the flow of breath.

3. Painting your upper body

(A used tennis ball is best, because it is a bit softer.)

Start on your back with feet flat on the floor, knees up with heels placed so that your legs feel easily supported in this position, as in #2. Your arms rest comfortably at your sides.

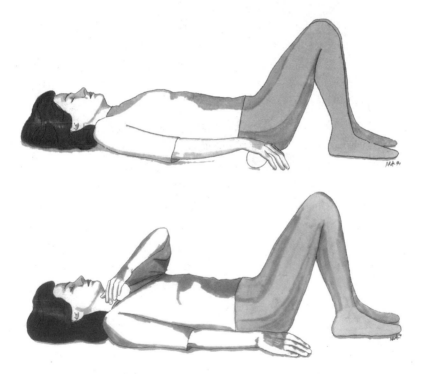

Figure 7.3 Painting Your Upper Body — two views.

Begin with the most comfortable side of your body. With the tennis ball under that hand, slowly and easily begin to roll your hand over the tennis ball on the floor, as if you were painting your whole hand with the ball. Wake up the whole surface of your hand, gently, just using the weight of your hand resting on the ball. Explore the palm of your hand, the back and between your fingers, allowing your hand to be soft and receptive to the touch of the ball. Remember spaces between the bones in your hand (the joints). Take time to rest periodically.

Gradually roll your wrist and arm on top of the ball. Explore the two bones of your lower arm and the space between them. Move up around your elbow, discovering the contours and possibilities of movement. Always be gentle with yourself, proceeding in a comfortable and easy way. From your elbow move to your upper arm, finding the one bone of your upper arm. Let your arm, head, and neck move freely with the movement of your hand. Find where your arm meets your shoulder, in a way that feels good, always listening to what your body would like to do today. Rest.

Now take the tennis ball in your opposite hand and gently roll it on top of your collar bone from your center out to your shoulder of the side you just explored. Roll the ball down the front of your sternum and out along your ribs. Each rib has a true joint with the sternum in the front and with your spine in the back, which allows the expansion and contraction of your breathing. Be aware of the spaces between your ribs. Come back to your starting position. Rest and observe how your chest and arms feel.

When you're ready. do the other side.

Sitting practices

Tools: Wooden chair or stool with a flat seat, a used tennis ball, non-binding clothes, relaxed jaw, and a curious mind.

These movements are best done beginning with the gentle stimulation of the skin with the tennis ball. The object is to do less and pay attention carefully to the feedback your body gives you. Rest often to allow your nervous system to assimilate the new information you are creating. Go through all the movements on one side of your body, stop and take time to feel the difference between the two sides, before doing the other side. Start with the side that is most comfortable that day. You can use these suggestions as preparation for more vigorous exercise, and as a springboard to explore how your body might like to move.

Your sitbones

Your sitbones – or ischial tuberosities – are the lowest points of your pelvis and architectural base of your spine (see Figure 7.5). Your hamstrings and most of the muscles of your inner thigh originate along the bottom ridge of your pelvis and sitbone. These are muscles that are chronically tight in most people. Attending to the origin of the muscles helps balance their level of activity. As you will see, knowing about your sitbones can also improve your relationship with your spine and upper body.

1. Clearing your sitbones

This practice is designed to ease and improve the support you receive from your pelvis when sitting. It is beneficial for your back, neck, shoulders, arms, and hands.

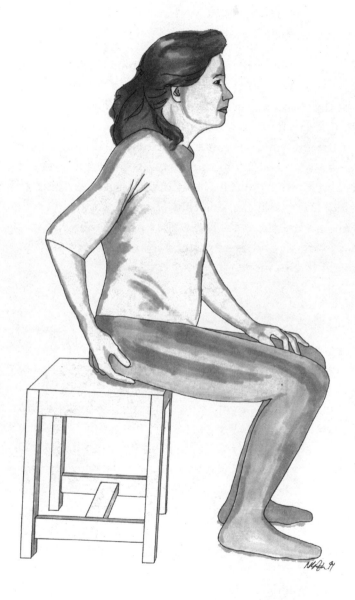

Figure 7.4 Clearing Your Sitbones.

Sit on a hard chair (Figure 7.4). Shift around a little, feeling for the two bottom points of your pelvis – your sitbones. Lean slightly to one side, lifting your hip. Reach underneath and touch your sitbone. Make friends with it, notice its shape, any tenderness, how the muscles around it feel. The hamstrings originate from the sitbones, so this is a good warm-up to lengthening those muscles which tend to be short on almost everyone.

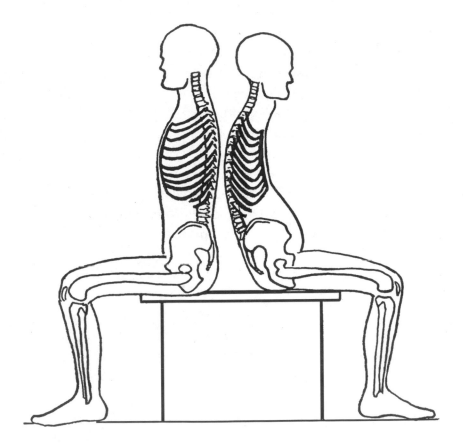

Figure 7.5 Sitbones and Spine— our inner architecture

Do this simple location exercise for several days. By getting acquainted with your sitbones, you will begin to reduce the muscle tension. When you feel ready, place the tennis ball behind your sitbone so that the ball displaces the muscles. Let your muscles drape over the ball. Feel the upward pressure of the ball. Image sending an opposite line of force back down through the ball into the floor, like a laser beam. Remove the ball and feel how your sitbone settles onto chair. Rest. Repeat this sequence in front, inside and outside of the sitbone. Sit on the ball only briefly – 20 to 30 seconds at the most. The time in between ball locations are the moments when you can really feel *how* you sit and release tension. Be sure to take time to feel the difference between your right and left sides after you have completed one side.

Awareness of your sitbones will help you develop more healthy and comfortable ways of sitting. Explore how you can move from that base. Place your hands in the crease of your pants on each side, in front. That is where your hip joints are located. Experiment bending from there, keeping the awareness of your sitbones. That is the place where you are meant to bend. It will protect your back to use those hinge-like joints. Play with reaching for something, first bending with a rounded back, then bending low at your hips. What is the difference? Play with how your spine can lengthen when you are aware of your hip joints, with your sitbones as the base and the back of your head (at the hairline) as the top of your spine. Use those two places as reference points in your walking and sitting.

Your feet

Your feet are your foundation for standing and moving. Most of us take them for granted, unless they start complaining.

Our feet are amazingly complex structures. Each of the 26 bones in the foot is contoured to form the arches of the foot (Figure 7.10). In addition, each bone of the toes and each metatarsal is arched, thus giving spring to our stride. The number of bones and joints allows for adjustment to our walking surface. However, in our modern world, most feet are locked away in stiff shoes that cramp their natural flexibility, often causing discomfort.

The way we use our feet can affect the relative comfort of our whole body. I spend a great deal of time with my clients focusing on how they carry their weight on their feet. Balanced support from the feet has increased confidence, created smoother strides and decreased hip and knee pain in many of my clients. Recall the illustration in Chapter Four (Figure 7.11) that shows the four points to be aware of, and play with for balance.

The next practice is an opportunity to gently explore your feet, one at a time. It can ease discomfort and feelings of fatigue when done with a patient and generous mind. As the organization of your foot improves you get better support to your ankle, knee and hip.

2. *Painting your foot*

Sit comfortably, aware of your sitbones, back easily elongated, the back of your head floating behind you. Roll a tennis ball under one foot, exploring the contours. Do this very gently, just stimulating the skin at first. Make contact with every part of the sole of your foot. Rest, foot flat on the floor. After a few minutes your can experiment using a little more pressure, if you like.

When you have completed one foot, rest. Observe the sensations of your foot, leg and whole body. Slowly stand and

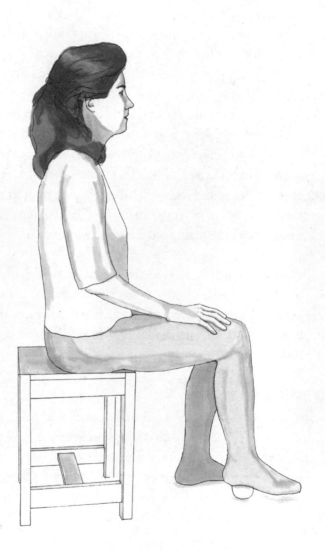

Figure 7.6 Painting Your Foot.

take a few steps. Compare how your feet feel. What is it like to walk now? When you are ready, do your other foot. When completed, rest again. Take time to see what happens. Slowly, mindfully walk. How do you feel?

Your thighs

Thighs are often overworked and under-appreciated. Some people tend to be very critical of this part of their anatomy. These elements of exertion and hostility can contribute to chronic tension in the thigh muscles, which in turn can not only limit your mobility, responsiveness and general posture, but also obscure the role that your femur plays in movement. The natural arch along the back of the bone can act as a propellant, bringing lightness to your stride. The following practice can help transform the experience of your thighs from a slab of meat to be reduced, to an active and supportive member of your movement team.

3. Fluffing your thigh

This is a simple tool you can use anywhere. It is beneficial to your feet, knees, hips and back. Sit as in #1 and #2. First, find your femur. Using curious and *kind* hands locate the bone through the mass of muscle. You may want to start at your knee, where the bone is very accessible and trace it back toward your hip. Remember the shape as you do this, the roundness, dips and arch.

Starting on the outer part of your thigh, near the hip, gently lift the muscles you can feel (a comfortable handful). Let your hands be friendly and supportive. After a few moments easily release the lift. Slowly and gently move down your thigh, toward your knee lifting and supporting the muscles, repeating in three or four places. As you become more sensi-

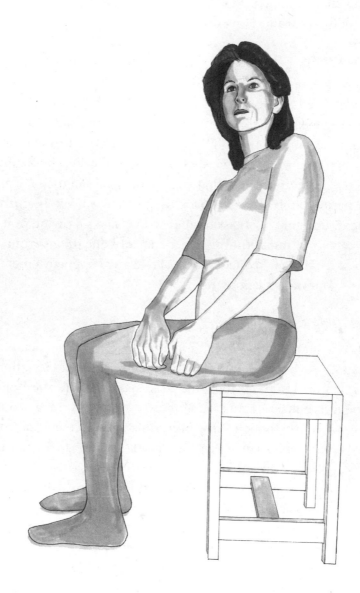

Figure 7.7 Fluffing Your Thigh

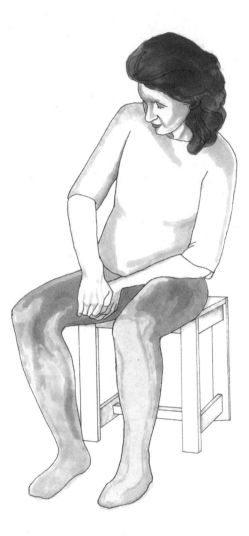

Figure 7.7b

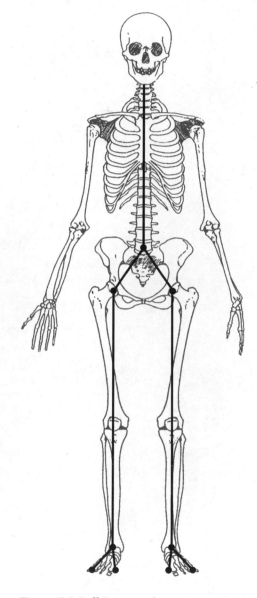

Figure 7.8 Full Support from Feet and Hips

tive, you will be able to feel your muscles relax as you support them. Hold the muscles gently, supporting them and encouraging them to let go. Then easily release the lift. Repeat this movement on the inner part of your thigh. Finally, using two hands, gently lift the group of muscles on the top of your thigh, starting close to the hip and moving toward the knee.

As you do this, be aware of not straining your upper body. I find it easiest to do the outer part of my thigh with straight arms, leaning away from lifted leg, using my weight to lift. With my inner thigh, I rest my forearm on the same-side leg. For example, my right forearm rests on my right thigh, using the right leg to help my arm create a lever as I reach under my left leg with both hands (Figure 7.7b). This arrangement helps to avoid overworking my arms or shoulders. Learning to catch the ways you strain yourself, and inventing new, easier ways, is a large part of the art of long-term comfort.

Walking basics: Form meets function

I have learned a great deal about walking, from myself and my clients. Here are some basic ideas to keep in mind for improving your gait. I focus on feet and hips because if the foot/hip relationship is good, stress is reduced in the knees and spine.

1. Your hip joints are only as far apart as your ears. Therefore, you get very central support for your upper body from your pelvis. This support forms an inverted Y, carrying the support from your feet and legs, to your hip joints and up into your spine (Figure 7.8).

2. The back of your femur is arched to facilitate an easy forward swing when walking. Feel the arch of your femur easily propelling your leg from behind like a wheel as you move forward (Figure 7.9). Direct your knees straight ahead.

3. The bones of your feet are arched, adding spring to the arch of your femur. You can use your toes, remembering the arched bones, to push off with adding spring and momentum in standing up, walking and climbing. This avoids overworking the knees and hip muscles (Figure

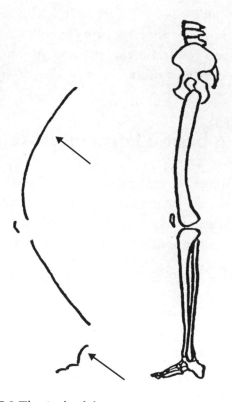

Figure 7.9 The Arch of the Femur - side view of left leg.

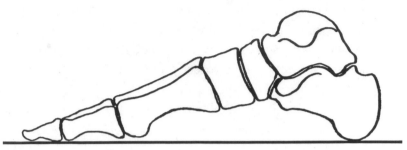

Figure 7.10 Arches in Bones of the Foot - view of inner arch of right foot.

7.10). Flexible soled shoes are very important to allow freedom of movement of the toes and arch in the foot.

4. The shape of your foot provides a broad base of support – remember the four weight-bearing points. Balanced placement of your heel stabilizes your leg (Figure 7.11).

5. Keep your strides of equal length.

6. Listen to your walk…keep your footsteps quiet and balanced.

7. Allow the back of your head to float behind you and your spine to easily lift (see Figure 4.6).

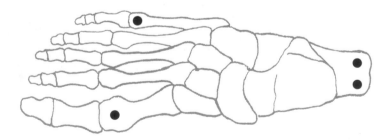

Figure 7.11 Stability of the Foot.

One of Newton's basic laws of physics is that "for every action there is an equal and opposite re-action." In other words, every time you step down, an equal force is carried *up through your body*. This force is most direct and efficient when your body is well aligned. The seven points listed above will prepare you to feel the lift from your feet, into your hips and up your spine, as described in #1, propelling you forward and up. When you feel this, you earn your ph.d. in movement awareness! Bone density is stimulated by weight bearing activity.[2] It is likely that improved alignment carries that benefit through the body more completely.

Other things to play with

1. Rehearse changes of position in your mind before you do them. Imagining your movement first prepares the nervous system, muscles and bones for the action. During recovery it is easy to move too quickly, without thinking, and tweak yourself. Learning to move consciously will always benefit you. Before you move, feel and see the easiest, most efficient way to accomplish the movement. Feel yourself doing it several times before you actually move, imagining with your body. This rehearsal process is very useful when changing positions, in which the transition can be uncomfortable, sitting to standing, for example. Take your time, be patient and allow yourself to adjust to the new position. Be open to the possibility that you *can* move comfortably.

2. Remember to care for the joints neighboring any area of difficulty. When one joint is hurt or immobilized, your other joints and limbs adjust by moving in new, some-

times odd ways. This can create other discomfort and potential future problems. For example, my left hip was the one operated on. To compensate for slight limitation in my ability to rotate from my hip, my left knee has exaggerated its natural range of movement for many years, weakening it slightly. In addition, my right leg, which I depended on so heavily before I learned to balance my walk, tends to be more tense and muscle bound. I take special care to keep those overworked places comfortable, and continue to improve the use of my left hip, so that it will pick up its rightful responsibilities.

3. Notice your pleasure, as well as your pain. Become aware of what parts of your body feel *good*. Learn from those places! What is a "good" feeling? How does it get there? Can the goodness be expanded? Frank Wildman Ph.D., Feldenkrais trainer, has developed a pleasure/pain scale which instructs the student to find two pleasurable associations with their body for every pain noted.[3] Try this out. Make up your own questions. Discover everything you can about your comfort; your discomfort has gotten the bulk of attention, I'll bet.

4. Move to your favorite music. Allow the music into your body. Feel how your body would like to move. Move with lightness. Let go of your ideas about how you should move. Enjoy.

5. If you have a pain, listen to it. How does it sound? Hum or sing the tone you feel. Match the feeling in your body with sound. Imagine that the sound can come from the point of discomfort.

Conclusion

I have found movement awareness essential to my continuing comfort and mobility. Awareness allows me to use my body intelligently, both consciously and unconsciously. Simple practices like the ones in this chapter allow me to do more vigorous exercise comfortably, without hurting myself. Increased awareness can make exercise more fun and interesting, too. For example, when I swim I imagine all of my bones cutting through the water (a swimming skeleton!). This makes me laugh, allows me to check my alignment and often increases my stamina (via distraction? who knows!). My clients report similar experiences. Consistency is critical. We need to keep moving to maintain the vibrant brain-extremities relationships, as discussed in previous chapters. Our physical interaction with the environment is essential to our development and ongoing sense of self.

Chapter 8

Keeping Your Balance

Each patient carries his own doctor inside him. We are best when we give the doctor who resides within each patient a chance to go to work.

– Albert Schweitzer

MANY OF US DO NOT GET INSPIRED TO CARE FOR ourselves until after a crisis occurs. The approach to self-awareness and care discussed in this book will be useful in crisis and will become second nature during more peaceful times. Our body is our home and as every homeowner knows maintenance is an ongoing necessity: A preventative approach will avert problems in the future. I am only half-joking when I remind my clients that life is maintenance.

Challenges to maintenance

You may not get much encouragement for creative maintenance from the medical community. Most doctors are schooled to be pessimistic, because the focus of medical training is pathology. They are prone to scoffing at any approach they don't understand or have not personally experienced. This attitude may explain why 7 out of 10 respondents in the Harvard study of unconventional medical practices did not tell their M.D.'s about the alternative approaches they were using (see Chapter One). Unfortunately, this perpetuates doctors' ignorance of the benefits of alternative care.

Many doctors are as likely to discuss the worst case scenarios as they are to encourage their patients. One of my hip replacement clients was told by her doctor that her muscles resembled those of "a paraplegic" and that she should not expect improvement. Another was told, "You better get used to being crippled" by her surgeon in the recovery room. How can people muster the motivation needed to recover when the medical authority has said these kinds of things?

Words are powerful

There is significant evidence that patients hear and understand what is said when they are under anesthesia.[1] Words strike deeply into the unconscious of a person struggling to recover, hoping for a "normal" active future. Remarks made by health professionals can have powerful effects on the patient who looks to the authority figures for guidance, hope and healing, as illustrated by the following examples.

An intensive care nurse told me of an experience she had when she was part of a special program to improve post-operative care. As part of the program she accompanied her patients through surgery and was the primary care-giver afterwards. One of her patients had severe colon problems, with lower abdominal complications. After the planned colostomy a plastic surgeon was called in to reconstruct the patient's vagina and pelvic floor. The nurse observed the two surgeons carry on a lengthy discussion, over the patient, about the gravity of the patient's condition and how she would never have a normal life or be sexually active again. Following the surgery the patient became extremely depressed. She spoke to the nurse frequently about her poor chances for recovery and of having a normal sex life – something she never mentioned prior to surgery. She repeated verbatim the phrases the nurse had heard the doctors use in the operating room. The patient never recovered. Upon hearing of this book, the nurse felt it was important that this story be told.

Operating room conversation can be recalled and the effects modified by the patient under hypnosis. A surgeon and hypnotherapist I work with became interested in what is heard by anesthetized patients because of his own experience. Following surgery for a football injury in college, he began fearing that he had cancer. This gnawing fear carried on for many years. Well into his adulthood he met Leslie LeCron, whose pioneering work with hypnosis developed methods that permitted consistent break-through of the amnesia associated with anesthesia and experiences of very early life.[2] My friend asked LeCron to help him uncover the source of his fear of cancer. While under hypnosis, he recalled the operating room conversation in which the surgeon referred to a lump, and then said "Let's get out of here" without doing anything about the lump. His subconscious mind misinterpreted the surgeon's remarks to mean that he had cancer. (The nature of the subconscious is literal and child-like, thus causing many misunderstandings.) Uncovering this memory explained the fear and removed the mysterious cloud hanging over his life. This experience forged a lifelong interest in exploring how operating room discussion affects patients and a commitment to teaching surgeons and anesthesiologists of the importance of what they say and do.

Surgeons and anesthesiologists have a great opportunity to use the power of the subconscious for encouraging hope and health. Positive words can help the client believe in themselves and their inner resources. An orthopedic surgeon told me of his recent experiences in this area. During the past two years he has changed his approach to surgery. Prior to each operation he meets the patient, talks to them and holds their hand as they go under the anesthesia. During surgery he makes a point of talking about the strengths in their body and the good recovery he expects for them. He feels much happier in his work doing this and his patients respond well. Perhaps the most impressive thing he has noticed is the consistent and significant reduction in his patients' blood loss during surgery. Therefore, blood transfusions and overall stress to the body were reduced. This is a factor in health care just waiting to be exploited for good on a large scale.(See the Resources section in the back of the book for more information.)

Resistance

It is hard to change, even when the change is in our best interest, even when we want to change. Resistance is a normal reaction to any attempt to shift our habitual way of thinking and behaving. We humans are creatures of habit. Voices inside us say things like, "I can't do this..." or, "I don't want to change," or "I don't deserve better." These are the voices of pain, fear and depression. These voices believe they have been protecting us all these years and they don't want to expose us to perceived dangers. Originally these internal warnings may have been important for survival, as in the case of an abused child who would be attacked for questioning the status quo. To move on in adulthood we must release our old ways. The challenge is to step forward in spite of resistance.

Strong emotions may arise as we begin to change. Feelings of anger, sadness, self-punishing thoughts, discouragement, or less specific reactions of lethargy or agitation are all common. Any of these indicate that unfinished business from the past is interfering with your new agenda. Emotional discomfort shows you your growing edge, giving you an opportunity to look again at the past and form a new approach to the present. Working through your emotional blocks may be your greatest challenge.

There have been times in my personal work when I could barely stand to notice the feelings in my body, because when I did there was more emotional pain than I wanted to feel. For example, for more than a year after my divorce I avoided my self-care routine of sensory awareness and movement. Whenever I began to increase my body awareness I would collapse in tears. Sometimes I could allow myself to stay with the pain, which manifested physically as a deep ache in my chest, in addition to my emotions. Other times I could not stand the pain, so I would shut my self off, even though I knew that the only way out was through it. With time and much personal work my sadness dissipated, although I am still caught by surprise sometimes when it re-emerges.

When there has been physical disability similar avoidance can arise from the pain and disbelief that things can change for the better. This is the nature of grief, it moves in cycles.

Grief is a natural reaction to loss of a loved one, physical abilities, or any aspect of one's life. Compassion, patience and devotion to your healing process will bring light into these times of darkness.

Our bodies process our emotional experiences from birth. The processing stops when we block our feelings, which in turn get stuck in our body. Beginning a practice of quiet and attentive self-care allows these memories to surface, which is sometimes daunting, but always healing. Any number of feelings can arise, especially when there has been a history of physical illness, trauma or abuse. While allowing the feelings to surface, it is important to remember that those feelings come from the past: that was then, this is now. The present is different, with new possibilities.

We all have a natural pull to stick with what is familiar. That way we don't have to go to the trouble of meeting the challenge of going into the unknown, or worrying about the success of our new way. The devil's advocate asks, "Will the new approach be better than the past?" We cannot know for certain. What is known, is that our old ways don't work anymore. The old way of outmoded behavior says "YOU CANNOT CHANGE!" To move on in our lives we must have the spirit to stand up and say "Yes, I can." As the poet Rilke suggests, "Perhaps all the dragons in our lives are princesses who are only waiting to see us act, just once, with beauty and courage."[3]

Curiosity: Self as laboratory

The ingredients for successful maintenance are curiosity, patience and commitment. Curiosity leads to finding new options and orientations not before experienced. This most positive trait leads to creative solutions that may be completely original, perhaps uncovering the best answer for your situation. Be curious intellectually, emotionally and physically, and you will discover yourself in a new way. I believe we are all naturally curious, but many of us lose our joy of the quest when we are squelched by people or experiences that make us lose heart. For example, I have a friend who, at the age of four or five, was paid by his grandfather to stop asking questions, thus getting a strong message about curiosity. Allow your innocence and questioning to return and blossom.

Feed your mind

Any new situation includes puzzles and blank spaces that can be explored with beneficial results. When facing or recovering from surgery, it can be reassuring and inspiring to learn about your anatomy and the procedure involved. Consistently, my clients feel more confident when I explain how their body works and how they can help themselves by being more aware of specific elements of balance and movement. Knowledge increases our sense of power, which is so important when we have been physically vulnerable.

Many resources exist for obtaining medical information. Reference librarians at public libraries are a good place to start. Some hospitals offer public medical libraries, computer bulletin boards offer information searches and doctors are generally willing to answer questions when they are asked. The information is accessible when approached with a curious mind, rather than a mind that says, "Science! EEEK, I can't understand that!" Thoughtful reading and common sense will show you that you can increase your understanding.

126 • *Finding Your Balance*

Emotional questions

Many interesting questions arise when you examine the role of your disease in your life. For example, in considering my long-term recovery from hip surgery, I still ask myself: How can I support my own recovery? How well do I support myself emotionally and spiritually? Does my work truly support me? Do I have issues of support in my relationships? Will my leg support me? Can I stand up for myself? Asking these kinds of questions is very useful in understanding the dynamics of our affliction.

Questioning is a great opportunity to learn something new about yourself and to recognize an old pattern. Any insights should be received as a gift of understanding which opens new doors, **never** turned against yourself. Dr. Larry Dossey addresses the problem of self-blame with story and comments:

> *In the ninth Book of John, Jesus and the disciples encounter a man who has been blind since birth. The disciples are troubled and ask a very New Age question: "Who hath sinned, this man or his parents that he is born blind?" And Jesus said "No one has sinned that this man is born blind, but that the works of God should be made manifest through him."…This may outrage our sense of cosmic justice, but spiritual achievement and physical health do not always go hand in hand. Sometimes the wisdom of the world works the other way, and the sages and saints suffer more than the wicked. Therein lies a paradox and a mystery beyond our powers of scrutiny. And it is important to recognize this, because otherwise it becomes all to easy to fall prey to the trap of self-blame when illness strikes.*[4]

Many of us carry harsh critics inside us who jump at the chance to demean and demoralize us. These are the voices of fear: fear that we don't measure up, that we will hurt ourselves, that we are wrong and on and on. Use your increasing awareness to see yourself objectively and compassionately. You are a student of life and can learn and grow from any information.

An expansive orientation to our problem gives us more avenues for addressing the situation. Our language is filled with body metaphors, and our bodies very often act out those metaphors. We can see how these metaphors are expressed in our lives. A good example of this is the direct relationship I discovered between my increased physical balance and stability, and my ability to speak up, support myself and take action in my world.

Testing the water

I have always been inspired by the words of existentialist Søren Kierkegaard, "To venture causes anxiety, but not to venture is to lose one's self. And to venture, in the highest sense is precisely to be conscious of one's self." Increasing and exploring your awareness of your physical body gives you a whole new dimension of self-knowledge. When you have experienced physical pain in the past, the tendency is to avoid feeling your body or trying anything new. Here, trust in the healing process and in your body's integrity is needed. You need to make friends with your body. New things can be tried, gently and methodically, monitoring your comfort zone. Becoming more attuned to how you feel and how you move will help you to learn more comfortable ways of moving and being.

Every few years I try a new method of bodywork, movement, or awareness training to expand my range of experience and ideas. I delight in discovering some new ability or insight and as I go along I am coming to know myself better and better. I am forced to believe in my potential, because I always surprise myself. I encourage you in this activity of thoughtful exploration. My hope is that you come to know yourself and trust your self-knowledge as much as you trust your doctor, so that if medical choices are to be made you participate actively from a position of self-knowledge, trust and respect. You will develop a "gut" feeling about what is right for you.

Patience

The time following surgery or injury is delicate. There is the relief of getting through the operation. There is physical disorientation. Your body needs time to cleanse itself of medications which have interrupted your metabolic processes. There are many emotions you feel as you face life with a body that has been modified in a matter of a few hours. Learn to listen and respect your inner needs (physical and emotional), rather than forcing your will. Do not listen to external ideas about how you "should" behave. Recovery is a wonderful opportunity to learn more about yourself and to lay the foundation for new self-support habits. Honor your own rhythm. Learn to observe and appreciate the subtleties of your body. Your life has changed and this is a call to know yourself anew.

New concerns about physical stability may appear after surgery or injury. Old fears become exacerbated due to the temporary, yet very real, lack of physical strength, coordination and balance. Orthopedic patients learning to walk again face these fears daily, restricting their freedom of movement. These concerns should not be ignored during recovery. Routinely, patients are given excellent medical treatment with no attention paid to how the physical interventions affect the person's emotional life.

Heart surgery, for instance, is tremendously invasive: one's chest is literally "cracked" open, in the medical jargon. Yet none of the heart patients I have spoken with has received any sort of acknowledgment of the emotional importance of the surgical site: their heart, their physical and emotional core. One patient, a doctor, was discovered by his sister holding a pillow to his chest and sucking his thumb shortly after bypass surgery. His feelings were never talked about and he later denied what his sister had seen. Where did his feelings go? My clinical and personal experience has shown me that suppressed feelings tighten the muscles around the area that has been operated on, forming a protective "armor" which restricts movement, and by extension, circulation. This leads me to be concerned about a heart patient whose chest continues to be held still, in a repressed emotional state.

The myth of weakness

When we have health difficulties we tend to view our symptoms as weaknesses. We go to experts on the physical body, expect them to "fix" us. We push ourselves to "bounce back." This is the nature of the conventional western approach to medical care. Weakness is to be eradicated, conquered in our western world view. Much as we fight against it, we are creatures of the natural world and in nature the cycles of regeneration and renewal cannot be rushed.

I worked with a knee replacement client whose knee had swollen terribly after her surgery. She called me because her doctor gave her no useful suggestions. In the course of our initial interview she said she had been doing her physical therapy exercises three hours a day, far more than what was prescribed. She assumed that more was better. No one else had asked her about the level of her activity. I suggested that she cut back to her original instructions and pay attention to what made her knee feel better. Within a week her pain and swelling decreased. As she became more aware and gentle with herself her comfort improved. Whenever she became impatient and harsh with herself her progress slowed.

Symptoms of weakness or tenderness are valuable messengers showing us where we need support and sustenance. A symptom is the body's call for attention to self, for rest, greater care, awareness in movement, or other possibilities. When a friend referred to his body as the "weak link" in his tired, over-stressed state. I corrected him, "your body is the *smart* link." Your body will stop you when you are too unaware to stop and listen to yourself. It is intelligent to take a break before you hurt yourself seriously, physically, emotionally and/or spiritually. Your body calls you to pause and reflect. Again, the key to continued comfort and successful maintenance is to heed the communication from your physical self.

Commitment

This book asks you to care for yourself and to make the kind of commitment to your health that you would make to your beloved. Staying healthy, body, mind and heart, is as de-

manding as the deepest emotional relationship and as rewarding. Participating in your health puts you in touch with
the divine: Creation.

This commitment to self calls upon you to take responsibility for your whole life. The doctor is a mechanic who can give
you structural help, but you must learn to drive wisely. You
have the opportunity to discover your strengths and build
your wellness using your tools of awareness, creativity and
courage.

You must train with the dedication of an athlete for meaningful success. Some days you may feel achy, have "more important" things to do, or just feel lazy. Everyone is
occasionally faced with the "stick-in-the-mud" syndrome.
This is where your commitment to yourself is critical. It takes
discipline to develop new habits and it may take time to feel
the benefits. The trick is to keep at it regularly, be it meditation, exercise or other self-awareness methods. You will find
these new ways are worth the effort. Your world will expand
with your awareness.

Rewards

Increasing physical comfort, peace of mind and the ability to
solve your own problems are among the rewards of developing a practice of self-awareness and care. My personal and
professional experience confirms the benefits of taking time
to recognize your vulnerabilities, strengths and capacity to
help yourself. Two innovative programs in the medical community demonstrate that the principles of active self-care
work on a large scale.

In 1979 the Stanford University Arthritis Clinic began offering self-care classes for people with arthritis. These classes
emphasize three concepts:

1. Each person with arthritis is different. There is no one treatment that is right for everyone.

2. There are a number of things people can do to feel better. These things will not cure most forms of arthritis, but they will help to relieve pain, maintain or increase mobility, and prevent deformity.

3. With knowledge, each individual is the best judge of which self-management techniques are best for him or her.[5]

The Arthritis Self-Help Book by Doctors Lorig and Fries describes this program, which includes education on how best to exercise, information regarding relaxation, nutrition, problem-solving, pain control and other self-management strategies. As of 1990, over 100,000 people had followed this program. Controlled studies showed that, "People who become good arthritis self-managers have less pain and are more active than those people who feel there is nothing they can do for themselves." This program finds it is never too late to start: Their oldest student was *100* years old when she first came to class. The clinical researchers caution that self-management is not a quick cure; remember, your problems did not develop overnight. "It is a way of life to be practiced every day for the rest of your life." [6]

Dr. Dean Ornish's Program for Reversing Heart Disease, presents an ambitious program of diet, exercise, support groups and stress management through meditation and yoga. In the first year of research, 82% of Dr. Ornish's patients showed an overall reversal of coronary artery disease. Consistent results like these prompted the insurance giant, Mutual of Omaha, to cover costs for subscribers participating in this treatment program. This is one of the first times the insurance industry has sponsored an alternative medical program that uses methods not taught in traditional medical school curricula. (Limited coverage of chiropractic and acupuncture is available through some carriers.) Ornish's use of the mind/body approaches of meditation and yoga, which have been demonstrated to be essential for his program's overall success, is significant. The acceptance and recognition of this program is a ground-breaking event in the world of health care. It is an affirmation of the principles put forth in this book and throughout the community of alternative health care providers.

Conclusion: New definition of healing

"Every thought, act and feeling is health creating or health destroying...the creation of health is an all pervasive phenomenon."

— Dr. William Stewart
Medical Director,
Program in Medicine
and Philosophy,
California Pacific Medical Center.

The conventional expectation of medical treatment is that it will "make the symptoms disappear," hopefully, forever. The medical system attempts to cure symptoms by external methods, leaving the patient to be a passive observer of technical wizardry. Quality of life is often sacrificed in the struggle to eradicate "the problem." Anyone who has been close to this experience is familiar with the loss of self in the face of this approach.

"Healing" comes from the root "to make whole." It is an interactive process; patient, health care providers and supportive family and friends working together. Healing may not be the same as cure, but it can be richer, more fulfilling and more sustaining because it is built from within, using our own strengths and insights. Each of us hopes we never feel pain, fear or depression again. The truth is that we must confront and dissolve our patterns of pain and self-restriction over and over throughout our lives. The good news is that with active awareness we can greet the cycle with increasing competency, creating an ascending spiral of understanding and resiliency. Therefore, healing, rather than a superficial fix, is a deep transformation. The process of health depends on the comprehensive action to balance all of the resources of this self of ours: physical, intellectual, emotional and spiritual.

Chapter 9

Nourishment

Everyone who is seriously involved
in the pursuit of science becomes convinced
that a Spirit is manifest in the Laws of the Universe
– a spirit vastly superior to that of man,
and one in the face of which we,
with our modest powers, must feel humble.

– Albert Einstein

THE ESSENTIAL ELEMENT OF MY CONTINUED IM-
PROVEMENT, and the motivation for my professional practice, is my growing experience of the
physical as spiritual. Spiritual defined as "personal
awarenesses of dimensions of existence which extend
beyond the physical domain but also encompass the
physical."[1] What is commonly thought of as physical
is also non-physical. *We must attend to both to main-*

tain balance. This is an evolving realization for me, beginning with the first therapeutic massage I received, which opened me to an altered state of awareness. The refinement and deepening of this experience of unity continues. Just as science is now proving that there is no separation between body and mind, I experience that my bodymind is also spirit and that my spirit is not separate from a larger source.

This is not a new idea. Organized religions have long called the body "the temple of the soul," but practice of this truth has been muted in recent times. We live in a world dominated by the intellectual, puritan ethic "don't feel," rendering life barren, crippled and isolated. If we accept that ethic, we are left without vibrance, without the joy found in dance of body and spirit. The dryness of the intellect calls out to be balanced, *sweetened* by the nectars of the soul.

I am compelled by the grace I experience watching my clients' healing processes. The following is an example of the moments of wonder I see in my practice:

A client was doing a simple movement as I described the sequence and layers of skin, tissue and bone that were being affected by the movement. As always I encouraged a meditative focus. In a voice filled with awe, the client whispered, *"It's like looking at the creation of Being, through the eyes of Being."*

This sense of the miraculous in simple awareness is deeply nourishing.

I believe this sense of nourishment has a great deal to do with the experience of the Divine. Aldous Huxley defined spirituality as "the art of achieving oneness with God." It is at once deeply personal and universal. There is a sense of inner sustenance and interconnectedness; awe at the magnitude, yet peace in the simplicity – like the quiet power of a sunset. This sense of expanded being creates a container to hold my life's challenges. This container gives me the courage to believe new things are possible; that the present and future can be different from the difficulties of the past. The container encourages me to trust the unfolding of my life.

Acceptance of Divine Order has allowed me to quell the war of fear and denial within me. It has taught me to step back and learn from myself and those around me. I feel more a part of nature and more compassion for the world around me. We cannot predict what life will hand us, but we can chose how we respond. I have discovered that the solutions are most often within, when time is taken to listen. We all have life lessons that are beyond our limited understanding; they create the great mystery of life. Yet, we can participate and expand our possibilities. The more I can accept life's challenge to stretch and grow, the more peace I experience, the more I am able to find my balance.

Footnotes

Chapter One

1. See discussion of Elsa Gindler and her work in *Sensory Awareness*, by Charles Brooks, Felix Morrow, Great Neck, New York, 1986. Pages 229–233.

2. Bersin, David. "An Interview with Gerda Alexander," in *Somatics*, Autumn/Winter, 1983. Pages 4–10.

3. Juhan, Deane. *Job 's Body: A Handbook for Bodywork*. Station Hill Press,In., Barrytown, New York, 1987. Page xxx.

4. Eisenberg, D., Kessler, R., Foster, C., et al. "Unconventional Medicine in the United States," *The New England Journal of Medicine*, 328:(January 28), 1993. Pages 246–252.

5. Chopra, "Timeless Mind, Ageless Body" in *Noetic Sciences Review*, Winter 1993. Page 18.

6. Pert, Candace. "The Material Basis for Emotions," in *The Whole Earth Review*, Summer, 1988. Pages 106–111.

Chapter Two

1. Excellent discussions of state-dependant-learning can be found in Cheek, David. *Hypnosis: The Application of Ideomotor Techniques*, W. W. Norton & Company, Inc. New York, 1993 and Rossi, Ernest. *The Psychobiology of Mind-Body Healing*. W. W. Norton & Company Inc., New York, 1986.

2. Goleman, Daniel. "The Experience of Touch: Research Points of a Critical Role," in *The New York Times*, 2/2/ 1988, C1.

Chapter Three

1. I Corinthians, 13. *The Bible,* King James Edition.

2. See discussion of love in Estes, Clarissa Pinkola. *Women Who Run With the Wolves.*Ballantine Books, New York, 1992. This quote on page 142.

3. Cousins, Norman. *Head First: The Biology of Hope.* E.P.Dutton, New York, 1989. Page 36.

Chapter Four

1. Linn, B., Linn, M., & Klimas, N., "Effects of Stress on Surgical Outcome," in *Advances,* 6(2) 1990. Page 22.

2. Kabat-Zinn, Jon. *Full Catastrophe Living: Using the Wisdom of Your Body and Mind to Face Stress, Pain and Illness.* Delta, New York, 1990. Pages 283–319.

3. Hall, Stephen, "A Molecular Code Links Emotions, Mind and Health," *Smithsonian.* June 1989. Page 65.

4. Merzenich, M., Recanzone, G., Jenkins W., Allard, T., & Nudo, R. "Cortical Representational Plasicity," in Rakic & Singer, (Eds.). *Neurobiology of the Neocortex.* Dahlem Workshop on Neurobiology of the Neocortex, Berlin, 1987. Page 47.

5. Feldenkrais, Moshe. *Awareness Through Movement.* Harper & Row, New York, 1977.

6. Stein, R., Brucker, B. & Ayyar D., "Motor units in incomplete spianla cord injury: electrical activity, contractile properties ant the effects of Biofeedback," *Journal of Neurology, Neurosurgery and Psychiatry.* 1990 October 53(10). Pages 880–885.

A more accessible discussion of Brucker and associates' work is available in a collection of popular articles which can be obtained from The Biofeedback Laboratory at the

Department of Orthopedics and Rehabilitation, University of Miami School of Medicine, P.O. Box 016960, Miami, Florida, 33101.

7. Suthers, Roderick & Gallant, Roy. *Biology: A Behavioral View.* Xerox College Publishing, Lexington, Massachusetts, 1973. Page 492.

Chapter Five

1. Cannon, Walter. *Bodily Changes in Pain, Fear and Rage*, D. Appleton-Century Company Inc., New York, 1934.

2. Waldholtz, Michael. "Mapping the Mind: Panic Pathway," in *The Wall Street Journal*, CXXIX:1-A8 (September 29) 1993. Page A8.

3. It is beyond the scope of this book to provide acomplete discussion of the current research on depression. I refer the interested reader to Wilner 's book for a more extensive examinataion of the subject: Willner, Paul. *Depression - A Psychobiological Syntheis.* John Wiley & Sons, New York, 1985.

4. Kabat-Zinn, Ibid. Pages 289–290.

Chapter Six

1. Information regarding the Rosen Method is available from the Rosen Method Professional Association, 2550 Shattuck Avenue, Box 49, Berkeley, CA, 94704.

2. See Rowan, John. *Subpersonalities.* Routledge, New York, 1990, for a good discussion of this broad view of personality theory.

3. If you are interested in further readings on meditation there are many fine sources available. I suggest starting with David Harp's, The Three Minute Meditator, or Jon Kabat-Zinn 's, Full Catastrophe Living. For a rich discussion of long-

term meditation practice I recommend <u>A Path with Heart</u>, by Jack Kornfield.

4. Achterberg, Jeanne. *Imagery in Healing*. Shambala Publications Inc., Boston, 1985. Pages 115–16.

5. Langer, Ellen. *Mindfulness*. Addison-Wesley Publishing Inc., New York, 1989. Page 62.

Chapter Seven

1. Eutony movments are discussed in Alexander, Gerda. *Eutony: The Holistic Discovery of the Total Person.* Felix Morrow, Great Neck, New York, 1985 and Lindell, Lucy. *The Sensual Body*. Simon and Schuster, London, 1987. Pages 112–123.

2. McIlwain, Harris, Bruce, D., Silverfield, J. & Burnette, M. *Osteoporosis: Prevention, Management, Treament.* John Wiley & Sons, New York, 1988. Page 22.

3. Wildman, Frank. "Pleasure," in *The Feldenkrais Journal,* 6:(Winter) 1991. Page 40.

Chapter Eight

1. Cheek, David. *Hypnosis: The Application of Ideomotor Techniques,* W. W. Norton & Company, Inc. New York, 1993.

2. Cheek, David and Le Cron, Leslie. *Clinical Hypnotherapy*, Grune & Stratton, New York, 1968.

3. Rilke, Rainer Maria, translated by Stephen Mitchell. *Letters to a Young Poet*. Vintage Books, Random House, New York, 1986. Page 92.

4. Dossey, Larry. "Healing and Prayer: The Power of Paradox and Mystery," in *Noetic Sciences Review*, 28:(Winter) 1993. Page 25.

5. Lorig, Kate and Fries, James. *The Arthritis Helpbook.* (Third Edition) Addison Westley Publishing Company, Inc. Reading, Massachusetts, 1990. Pages xiii–xiv.

6. Ibid. page xiv.

Chapter Nine

1. Benor, Daniel & Benor, Rita. "Spiritual Healing Assuming the Spiritual is Real," in *Advances*, 9(4):(Fall) 1993. Page 22.

Resources

To order *Finding Your Balance*, or for information about audio and video tapes based on the material in this book you may contact:

The Institute of Orthopedic Psychology
P. O. Box 3178
Sausalito, CA 96966
800/297-1197

Bodywork

I have listed the methods which I have experienced and recommend. Trained practitioners can be found in many communities by contacting the professional organizations listed below. Each method is gentle enough for people who have recently had surgery or prefer less invasive approaches. These methods are at once subtle and very beneficial. Always communicate clearly with your practitioner for the best results.

Accupressure:

The Acupressure Institute
1533 Shattuck Avenue

Berkeley, CA 94706
510-845-1059

*Feldenkrais Functional Integration and Awareness
Through Movement:*

Feldenkrais Guild
706 Ellsworth Street, P.O. Box 489
Albany Oregon 97321-0143
800/775-2118

Rosen Method Bodywork and Movement:

Rosen Method Professional Association
2550 Shattuck Ave. Box 49
Berkeley, CA. 94704
415/644-4166

Books

If you have enjoyed this book and want more information and inspiration I strongly recommend these books.

*Achterberg, Jeanne, Dossey, Barbara and Kolkmeier, Leslie. *Rituals of Healing*. Bantam Books, New York, 1994.

Anderson, Nancy. *Work With Passion*. New World Library, San Rafael, CA, 1984, revised edition 1995.

Chopra, Deepak. *Ageless Body, Timeless Mind*. Crown Books, New York, 1993. (Chopra has written several excellent books, I recommend any one of them.)

Field, Joannna. *A Life of One's Own* (Reprint). Putnam Publishing Group, New York, 1981.

*Goleman, Daniel & Gurin, Joel (Eds.). *Mind Body Medicine: How to Use Your Mind for Better Health*. Consumer Reports Books, New York, 1993.

Kabat-Zinn, Jon. *Full Catastrophe Living: Using the Wisdom of Your Body and Mind to Face Stress, Pain and Illness*. Delta, New York, 1990.

Kornfield, Jack. *A Path With Heart*. Bantam Books, New York, 1993.

Sacks, Oliver. *A Leg to Stand On* (Revised Edition). Picador, London, 1991.

* *These books are especially useful in the preparation for surgery and dealing with operating room conversation.*

Bibliography

Achterberg, Jeanne. *Imagery in Healing*. Shambala Publications Inc., Boston, 1985.

Achterberg, Jeanne, Dossey, Barbara and Kolkmeier, Leslie. *Rituals of Healing*. Bantam Books, New York, 1994.

Alexander, Gerda. *Eutony: The Holistic Discovery of the Total Person*. Felix Morrow, Great Neck, New York, 1985.

Anderson, Nancy. *Work With Passion*. New World Library, San Rafael, CA, 1984, revised edition 1995.

Brooks, Charles. *Sensory Awareness*. Felix Morrow, Great Neck, New York, 1986.

Chopra, Deepak, "Timeless Mind, Ageless Body," in *Noetic Sciences Review*, 28:16-21 (Winter) 1993.

Cousins, Norman. *Head First: The Biology of Hope*. E.P.Dutton, New York, 1989.

Dienstfrey, Harris. *Where the Mind Meets the Body*. HarperCollins, New York, 1991.

Douglas-Klotz, Neil. *Prayers of the Cosmos*. Harper & Row, San Francisco, 1990.

Fadiman, James. *Unlimit Your Life: Setting and Getting Goals*. Celestial Arts, Berkeley, California, 1989.

Field, Joannna. *A Life of One 's Own* (Reprint). Putnam Publishing Group, New York, 1981.

Garfield, Charles. *Peak Performers: the New Heroes of American Business*. Avon, New York, 1986.

Goleman, Daniel & Gurin, Joel (Eds.). *Mind Body Medicine: How to Use Your Mind for Better Health*. Consumer Reports Books, New York, 1993.

Harp, David. *The Three Minute Meditator*. mind's i press, S.F. 1987.

Kabat-Zinn, Jon. *Full Catastrophe Living: Using the Wisdom of Your Body and Mind to Face Stress, Pain and Illness*. Delta, New York, 1990.

Kornfield, Jack. *A Path With Heart*. Bantam Books, New York, 1993.

Langer, Ellen. *Mindfulness*. Addison-Wesley Publishing Inc., New York, 1989.

Lindell, Lucy. *The Sensual Body*. Simon and Schuster, London, 1987.

Lorig, Kate and Fries, James. *The Arthritis Helpbook*. (Third Edition) Addison Westley Publishing Company, Inc. Reading, Massachusetts, 1990.

Marieb, Elaine. *Human Anatomy and Physiology*. Benjamin/ Cummings Publishing Company Inc. 1989.

Montagu, Ashley.*Touching: The Human Significance of the Skin*. Columbia University Press, New York, 1971.

Moody, Raymond. *Life After Life*. Bantam Books, New York, 1975.

Ornish, Dean. *Doctor Dean Ornish 's Program for Reversing Heart Disease*. Random House, New York, 1990.

Perls, Fritz. *Gestalt Therapy Verbatum*. Real People Press, Lafayette, CA, 1969.

Perls, Fritz, Hefferline, Ralph, & Goodman, Paul. *Gestalt Therapy*. Bantam Books, New York, Third Printing 1980.

Sacks, Oliver. *A Leg to Stand On* (Revised Edition). Picador, London, 1991.

Schiffman, Muriel. *Self Therapy*. Self Therapy Press, Menlo Park CA, 1967.

------- *Gestalt Self Therapy*. Self Therapy Press, Menlo Park CA, 1971.

About the Author

Kate S. O'Shea, M.A. is the founder and director of the Institute of Orthopedic Psychology. Born with a dislocated hip, she underwent four major hip surgeries before the age of 14. Kate brings together her graduate education in psychology at the University of California, The Tavistock Institute of Human Behavior in London and Antioch University, with years of training in the field of bodymind awareness. She was among the first certified practitioners of the Rosen method of bodywork. Inspired by personal experience, she creates an approach to orthopedic conditions that is compassionate, precise and practical. Kate has worked with people in a variety of health education settings since 1975.

Kate would love to hear from her readers. Correspondence, book and tape orders, and inquiries for consultation can be addresssed in c/o Institute of Orthopedic Psychology, P.O. Box 3178, Sausalito, CA 94966. The number is 800 297-1197.

Index